A History of American Nursing

| TRENDS AND ERAS

Deborah M. Judd, MSN, FNP-C
Assistant Professor of Nursing
Weber State University
Ogden, Utah

Kathleen Sitzman, PhD, RN
Associate Professor of Nursing
Weber State University
Ogden, Utah

G. Megan Davis, MSLS
Health Sciences Librarian
Weber State University
Ogden, Utah

JONES AND BARTLETT PUBLISHERS
Sudbury, Massachusetts
BOSTON   TORONTO   LONDON   SINGAPORE

BP45

World Headquarters
Jones and Bartlett Publishers
40 Tall Pine Drive
Sudbury, MA 01776
978-443-5000
info@jbpub.com
www.jbpub.com

Jones and Bartlett Publishers Canada
6339 Ormindale Way
Mississauga, Ontario L5V 1J2
Canada

Jones and Bartlett Publishers International
Barb House, Barb Mews
London W6 7PA
United Kingdom

Jones and Bartlett's books and products are available through most bookstores and online booksellers. To contact Jones and Bartlett Publishers directly, call 800-832-0034, fax 978-443-8000, or visit our website www.jbpub.com.

Substantial discounts on bulk quantities of Jones and Bartlett's publications are available to corporations, professional associations, and other qualified organizations. For details and specific discount information, contact the special sales department at Jones and Bartlett via the above contact information or send an email to specialsales@jbpub.com.

The authors, editor, and publisher have made every effort to provide accurate information. However, they are not responsible for errors, omissions, or for any outcomes related to the use of the contents of this book and take no responsibility for the use of the products and procedures described. Treatments and side effects described in this book may not be applicable to all people; likewise, some people may require a dose or experience a side effect that is not described herein. Drugs and medical devices are discussed that may have limited availability controlled by the Food and Drug Administration (FDA) for use only in a research study or clinical trial. Research, clinical practice, and government regulations often change the accepted standard in this field. When consideration is being given to use of any drug in the clinical setting, the health care provider or reader is responsible for determining FDA status of the drug, reading the package insert, and reviewing prescribing information for the most up-to-date recommendations on dose, precautions, and contraindications, and determining the appropriate usage for the product. This is especially important in the case of drugs that are new or seldom used.

Production Credits

Publisher: Kevin Sullivan
Acquisitions Editor: Emily Ekle
Acquisitions Editor: Amy Sibley
Associate Editor: Patricia Donnelly
Editorial Assistant: Rachel Shuster
Production Assistant: Lisa Cerrone
Senior Marketing Manager: Barb Bartoszek

V.P., Manufacturing and Inventory Control: Therese Connell
Text Design and Composition: Shawn Girsberger
Cover Design: Kristin E. Parker
Photo Research Manager and Photographer: Kimberly Potvin
Printing and Binding: Malloy, Inc.
Cover Printing: Malloy, Inc.

Photographic credits and cover credits appear on page 249, which constitutes a continuation of the copyright page.

Library of Congress Cataloging-in-Publication Data
Judd, Deborah.
  A history of American nursing : trends and eras / Deborah Judd, Kathleen Sitzman, and G. Megan Davis
        p. ; cm.
  Includes bibliographical references and index.
  ISBN 978-0-7637-5951-3 (pbk.)
  1. Nursing—United States—History. I. Sitzman, Kathleen. II. Davis, Megan, 1978- III. Title.
  [DNLM: 1. History of Nursing—United States. 2. History, 20th Century—United States. 3. History, Modern 1601—United States. WY 11 AA1 S623h 2009]

RT4.J83 2009
610.730973—dc22

2008044967

6048

Printed in the United States of America
13 12 11 10 09   10 9 8 7 6 5 4 3 2

7/7/10

Contents

Preface

BASIC UNDERSTANDING OF NURSING HISTORY is essential to the development of a mature perception and appreciation of the nursing profession. Unfortunately, the heavy content load associated with BSN curriculum leaves a limited amount of time in which to study nursing history, making a comprehensive, time-intensive approach impractical. In response to this problem, this text takes a streamlined yet inclusive approach, focusing on historical trends in nursing that emerged in the United States from the 1600s to the present. It is designed to engage instructors and students in an exploration of events, issues, and advances related to nursing and associated with specific time periods in American history. The aim is to inspire excitement and interest while respecting the need to avoid the time and content overload so often present in BSN nursing curriculum.

The text is succinct enough that other texts or readings may be easily coupled with it to deepen study in areas specific to curriculum or course needs or instructor interests. (Additional resources are available through the publisher's catalog page for this book [**http://www.jbpub.com/catalog/9780763759513/**]. The catalog page may also be accessed by visiting **http://www.jbpub.com** and searching the keyword "Judd".) There is a focus on the relevance of *past* nursing history to *current* nursing practice, providing an opportunity for students and instructors to explore personal and professional meanings and applications of yesterday's events to today's world. Students and instructors are also invited to ponder ideas for future exploration related to historical trends in nursing.

Knowledge of nursing history encourages students to cultivate pride in the fact that they belong to a dynamic profession whose members have contributed immensely to the social fabric of this nation. Exploration of nursing's rich past also serves to remind today's students that their actions will determine future nursing history and empowers them to take an active role in creating a commendable future.

Kathleen Sitzman, PhD, RN

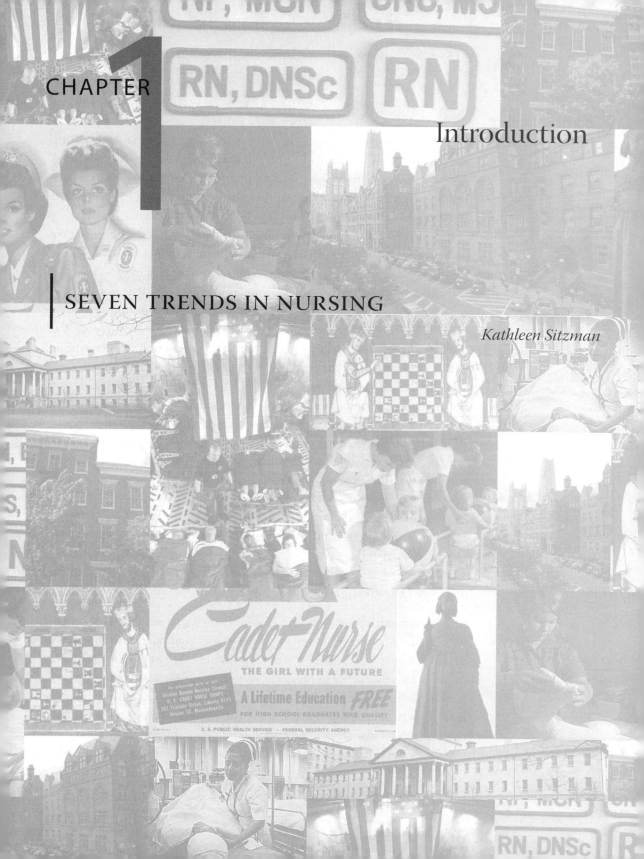

CHAPTER 1

Introduction

SEVEN TRENDS IN NURSING

Kathleen Sitzman

WHEN NURSING STUDENTS LEARN THAT they will be required to study nursing history, they often question the usefulness of such an endeavor, preferring instead to focus on learning information related to the mechanics of current clinical practice. It is sometimes difficult to envision how something that happened 100, 50, or even 10 years ago could possibly be relevant to the continually changing and fast-paced world of nursing today. In truth, past events (even some that occurred hundreds of years ago), still exert a profound influence on current nursing practice, particularly in relation to seven basic trends associated with image, education, advancement in practice, war, workforce issues, licensure/regulation, and research. It is essential to remember that these seven trends influence each other and are intertwined; however, there are unique aspects related to each trend that warrant separate discussion in the pursuit of elemental understanding within the context of the whole.

The organization and presentation of information in this text is based on the premise that spotlighting these seven trends in relation to specific time periods (eras) will enhance awareness of key forces that continually shape American nursing through time. This approach fosters professional growth and leadership grounded in knowledge of what has come before, thereby facilitating positive change towards a productive future during which past mistakes will hopefully not be repeated.

Explanations of the seven trends listed previously are provided below. Examining these trends in relation to the eras addressed in each chapter forms the basis of this text.

The Image of Nursing

Mass communication and entertainment that started with widespread use of the printing press in Europe in the 1600s and continued with the advent of radio, movies, television, and most recently, the Internet, have led to commonly held, generalized impressions related to nurses and the nursing profession. Contradictory images of nursing became popular during different eras, resulting in a composite and inconsistent public perception of American nurses. Popular public perception of nurses influences how nurses are treated by patients, other healthcare professionals, and the public. It also has an effect on how nurses perceive themselves and the profession, and how they treat each other in the workplace.

The Education of Nurses

Early nursing education was based on apprenticeship and observation. More formal methods of education emerged as a result of the work of nurse leaders in Europe and the United States. What began as an unregulated, informal, highly inconsistent endeavor grew into a systematic, consistent, regulated, academically rigorous pursuit that is required of all who wish to become professional nurses. General educational practices influence professionalism and consistency of care delivery. Level of education influences whether or not a profession has the training and infrastructure to develop its own knowledge base and then substantively interact within interdisciplinary teams consisting of other highly educated professionals.

Advances in Practice

For the purposes of this text, *advances in practice* refers to advances in healthcare technology and the development of new practice approaches/disciplines to effectively treat healthcare concerns. Technological advances through time have resulted in interventions that earlier healthcare providers could not imagine, for example antibiotics, insulin, ventilators, artificial hearts and limbs, organ transplants, intricate wound-care protocols, anesthesia, effective pain management, and genetic engineering. Technological advancements influence and (hopefully) improve outcomes and have resulted in perpetually fast-paced changes to nursing practice. New practice approaches/disciplines have been developed over time to address specific client concerns; for example, school nursing emerged in the early 1900s to meet the basic healthcare needs of lower income schoolchildren in industrialized cities who would otherwise not have the money to receive necessary medical care.

War and Its Effects on Nursing

The evolution of professional nursing in the United States is intricately tied to wartime activities. American nurses have consistently entered the armed forces when bidden and acted with bravery and honor wherever needed. Each war posed unique challenges and opportunities for nursing related to expanded professional roles and responsibilities. Innovative battle-field medical interventions have resulted in significant advances in emergency, trauma, and intensive care practices. Groundbreaking rehabilitative approaches for war-related injuries have led to advancements in prosthetics, psychiatric care, and neurological care. Cutting-edge treatments originally created to save and improve the lives of American soldiers have ultimately enhanced survival and quality of life for all Americans. Much of the technology that nurses routinely use today is the direct result of wartime.

Nursing Workforce Issues

Workforce issues related to supply and demand of qualified nurses have consistently emerged, sometimes related to an overabundance of nurses and more often connected to shortages. Other issues have concerned the employment of men, ethnic minorities, and racial minorities in nursing. Nursing began in the United States as primarily the work of Caucasian females; however, numbers of men and ethnic/racial minorities entering the nursing profession have steadily increased. Increased numbers of men and other minorities entering nursing have transformed workplace cultural/social dynamics from homogeneity to integration and variety. Workforce issues influence nursing practice on a daily basis, particularly during periods of shortage.

Licensure and Regulation

Early nursing in the United States was an informal endeavor. Anyone who felt knowledgeable about how to take care of others who were ill, injured, or in childbirth could assume the role of nurse and offer services for pay. As nursing education became more formalized and consistent, licensure and regulation issues came to the forefront, and all practicing nurses were eventually required to obtain and maintain licenses. As time went on, advanced practice nursing roles stimulated ongoing licensure/regulation debate around the issues of prescriptive authority and degree of autonomy in practice. The recent influx of foreign nurses wanting to work in the United States has prompted dialogue related to licensure/regulation of nurses who are not American citizens. Licensure/regulation laws set the tone for entry into different levels of nursing practice and ensure accountability of all professional nurses.

Nursing Research

Early nursing practice was based on tradition rather than systematic study of efficacy. Movement of nursing education into university settings stimulated research activities aimed at assessing effectiveness of nursing interventions and clarifying how nursing practices could be improved to support optimal client outcomes. Emergence of the widely accepted concept of evidence-based practice has resulted in increasingly dynamic knowledge development related to a wide range of nursing activities and disciplines. Continued advancement and refinement of the nursing knowledge base is an obligation of all professional nurses. BSNs provide questions/topics for inquiry and implement research findings at the clinical level. MSNs do all that BSNs do, plus assist in the creation and execution of research studies. Doctorally prepared RNs do all that BSNs and MSNs do, plus they create and manage all aspects of research studies. All RNs have the responsibility of disseminating results. Maintaining an adequate knowledge base that will support the growth and continued development of the nursing profession requires vigorous research activity at all levels of professional nursing.

How the Chapters in This Text Are Arranged

NURSING HISTORY UNFOLDED WITHIN LARGER sociopolitical climates. Each chapter begins with a brief overview of the general sociopolitical climate related to the era covered in that chapter. Exploration of how the seven trends discussed in this chapter manifested during that era follows. This text is a basic overview, with a focus on general trends and eras rather than examination of exhaustive historical information.

Timelines in Chapters 2 through 10 provide visual maps for key events; key people and their accomplishments are also briefly outlined at the beginning of these chapters. Topics for further exploration, discussion questions, book lists, and suggested key words/phrases for Internet exploration are provided at the end of the chapters to support and stimulate further study where time and interest permit.

◀ SUGGESTED READING

Andrist, L. C., Nicholas, P. K., & Wolf, K. A. (Eds.). (2006). *A history of nursing ideas.* Sudbury, MA: Jones and Bartlett.

Baer, E. D., D'Antonio, P., Rinker, S., & Lynaugh, J. E. (Eds.). (2002). *Enduring issues in American nursing*. New York: Springer.

Brinkley, A. (2003). *American history: A survey* (11th ed.). New York: McGraw-Hill.

Collins, G. (2003). *America's women: 400 years of dolls, drudges, helpmates, and heroines.* New York: William Morrow.

D'Antonio, P., Baer, E. D., Rinker, S. D., & Lynaugh, J. E. (Eds.). (2007). *Nurses' work: Issues across time and place.* New York: Springer.

Donahue, M. P. (1996). *Nursing: The finest art* (2nd ed.). St. Louis: Mosby.

Kalisch, P. A., & Kalisch, B. J. (2004). *American nursing: A history* (4th ed.). Philadelphia: Lippincott, Williams, & Wilkins.

Kerber, L. K., & DeHart, J. S. (1995). *Women's America: Refocusing the past* (4th ed.). New York: Oxford University Press.

Wolf, Z. R. (1988). *Nurses' work: The sacred and the profane.* Philadelphia: University of Pennsylvania Press.

CHAPTER 2

Nursing in the American Colonies from the 1600s to the 1700s

Past–1800 Nurses are generally male, or are sisters in a religious order

1500–1800 Hospitals are associated with religious organizations

1543
Andreas Vesalius
revolutionizes study of
human anatomy and
dissection

| 1600 | 1610 | 1620 | 1630 | 1640 | 1650 | 1660 | 1670 | 1680 | 1690 |

1600–1800 No formally trained nurses, but people in nursing roles include:
- Orderlies in mental hospitals
- Lay midwives
- Wetnurses
- Servitude caregivers
- Monks and sisters

1660–1800 • Significant bouts of infectious disease due to a lack of understanding of sanitation
  • Unhealthy individuals are cared for and die at home

1600–1850 Pesthouses and poorhouses are places for the sick to go to be isolated from the public

1618–1643 William Harvey studies and describes circulation

1618–1648 Thirty Years' War in Europe

THE INFLUENCE OF PAST IDEAS, TRADITIONS, AND TRENDS

Kathleen Sitzman

1770
Boston Massacre

1751
Pennsylvania Hospital
opened

1773
Boston Tea Party

1791
New York Hospital
opened

1700   1710   1720   1730   1740   1750   1760   1770   1780   1790   1800

1789
George Washington
elected first president
of the United States

1754–1763 French and Indian War

1765–1767 Two medical schools established in the U.S.

1775–1781 Revolutionary War

OUR NURSING HERITAGE: KEY PEOPLE

Ancient Civilizations contributed to health knowledge, they are not only key people but are key groups of people. Their ideas contributed to health care despite the scientific limitations of the time. These notions influence health care even into the 21st century.

Early Civilization	Illness associated with evil
	Gods determine life course/experiences
	Healing as an art: only certain individuals entitled to serve
	Community or family involved in rituals
Ancient Egyptian	Priests viewed as healers
	Practice of mummification and death rituals
	Organs separated from body and preserved
	Dental health a concern
	Sophisticated procedures done with limited technology
Middle Eastern	Concept of Yin and Yang
	Energy work
	Acupuncture
	Use of herbal medicines
Islamic	Concept that evil causes disease and suffering
	Principles based on Galen's and Hippocrates' application of the Four Humors to medicine
	Canon of medicine
	Noted minor differences in infectious diseases
	Chemistry advances: instillation, sublimation for medicines
Grecian	Aesculapius and his daughters: Hygeia, Meditrine, Panacea
	Aristotle: heart as the soul of body, vessels from heart
	Galen's concept of human anatomy
	Linked Empedocles to Four Humors, applied to medicine
	Hippocrates: father of medicine
	Role of Deaconesses: collection of alms, caring for the poor
Roman	Practices derived from Greek influence, Galen's influence
	Wealthy entitled to medical care, poor are not

Medieval Cultures	Emergence of hospitals: mostly for the poor, chronically ill Lay caregivers, both male and female
Early American	Traditional medicine of native tribes Health as a balance of life (person, nature, supernatural) Early settlers use poorhouses and home care Prevalent quackery, heroic cures, skepticism
Folk Culture	Based on cultural norms, passed between generations Idea that living plants and parts of organisms can heal Blood letting, leaches, potions
Order of Knighthood	Warrior caregivers: Templar Knights, While Knights
Monks	Healers who separated from society to serve society
Nuns or Sisters	Female healers in hospitals and poorhouses Sponsored and supported by certain religious organizations
Leopold Auenbrugger	Instituted percussion as an assessment technique
Robert Boyle	Father of modern medical chemistry Refuted Four Humors as basis of care
Vincent Chigarrigi	Proposed standards of care for the mentally ill
Lenardo Da Vinci	Anatomical representations of body Portrayed uterine environment and the fetus correctly
John Floyer	Created the "pulse watch" to check pulses
William Harvey	Scientific inquiry - anatomy/physiology Accurately described circulation of blood
John Hunter	Used simpler and safer techniques in operative procedures
Edward Jenner	Developed initial smallpox vaccination, principles applied to vaccination in use today
Athanasius Kircher	Used microscope to study microorganisms and their connection to disease
Giovanni Morgagni	Recognized disease comes from organ(s)
Thomas Sydenham	Theory that care should be based on a diagnosis
Anton van Leeuwenhoek	Discovered aspects of microbiology Described spermatozoa, bacteria, and protozoa

Sociopolitical Climate

URING THE 1600s AND 1700s, Colonial America was considered an outpost of Great Britain. The sociopolitical climate was influenced by steady European migrations to the colonies and preoccupation with the arduous business of forging a society that could adequately function without continual aid from Great Britain. Formal community-building activities and the creation of governing bodies were modeled after standards and practices in Great Britain; however cultural and religious norms varied widely due to the regional and ethnic diversity of the settlers. Expansion and development in the colonies during the 1600s and 1700s was accompanied by unrest related to the desire for autonomy and what was perceived as unfair taxation by Great Britain. Mounting discontent resulted in the beginning of the American Revolution in 1775 (Brinkley, 2003).

The Image of Nursing

HE IMAGE OF NURSES IN America during the 1600s and 1700s was synonymous with popular perceptions held in Great Britain and Europe because settlers understandably brought established attitudes and viewpoints with them to the colonies and then perpetuated them as time went on. Understanding the image of nursing in the American colonies requires a brief explanation of preceding conditions in Great Britain and Europe.

Beginning around 700 A.D. and continuing into the 1500s, most nursing care in Great Britain and Europe that was not provided by family members in the home was provided by monks and nuns in monastery wards as part of religious charity work. In these monastery wards, cleanliness and comfort were attended to and basic healing treatments of the day were administered. Ill and injured soldiers out in the battlefield received nursing care from knights who were assigned to provide such care when they were not engaged in battle. These

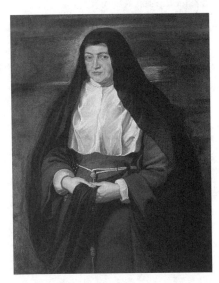

Isabella Clara Eugenia as a Poor Clare nun in 1625

esteemed and pious men and women who provided nursing care were viewed as altruistic and self-sacrificing (Donahue, 1996).

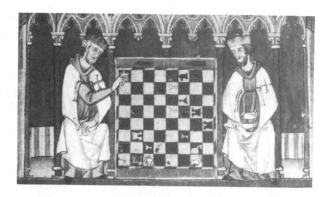

The Knights Templar playing chess

The Reformation (Protestant Revolt) began slowly in 1517 when Martin Luther, a disillusioned Catholic monk, publicly posted his 95 concerns (theses) about the Catholic Church on the Castle Church door. Inspired by the work of Martin Luther, Protestants (people who opposed the Catholic Church) continued to question the authority and practices of the Catholic Church until contention between the two erupted into an international conflict known as the Thirty Years' War that lasted from 1618 to 1648. During this time (known as the Reformation), most monastic institutions that provided care to the sick were destroyed or closed, which resulted in almost complete removal of men from nursing. Many nursing orders for nuns (women) were also eliminated. The few remaining religious orders that focused on caring for the sick were for women (nuns) only. The perception of nursing as women's work began at this time (Donahue, 1996).

The destruction and closures of monastery sick wards during the Reformation resulted in the creation of public hospitals where laywomen were expected to perform nursing care. Unlike monastery wards, which were generally considered to be clean, adequately supplied, and well-managed, public hospitals were filthy, chaotic, poorly appointed, disorganized, stench-filled buildings where patients went to die when they had no other alternatives. Most laywomen, who were not nuns and had not taken religious vows of service, charity, and poverty, were not willing to care for the sick in these deplorable public hospitals, and it was often difficult to secure adequate staffing. Judges in the legal system began giving prostitutes, publicly

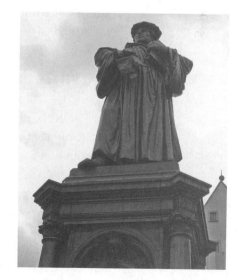

Martin Luther Statue, Eisleben, Lutherstadt, Saxony-Anhalt, Germany

intoxicated women, and poverty-stricken women the option of going to jail, going to the poorhouse, or working in the hospitals. Hospitals became full of nurses who were not trained, motivated, or qualified to care for the sick. These down-and-out nurses were known to steal from the patients, provide paid sexual favors for patients, and accept partial payment for their services in alcohol (Donahue, 1996; Kalisch & Kalisch, 2004). The image of nursing went from that of altruistic men and women selflessly caring for the sick to criminally inclined women either taking advantage of the sick at worst or providing incompetent care at best. During the 1600s and 1700s in the American colonies, healthcare practices and public perceptions of nursing closely resembled those in Great Britain (Kalisch & Kalisch, 2004).

The Education of Nurses

NURSES IN THE AMERICAN COLONIES during the 1600s and 1700s were not formally educated, relying instead on knowledge gained from personal experiences related to caring for ill, injured, or childbearing family members and friends. Colonial women inclined to do nursing work were often functionally illiterate, and for the few who could read, textbooks or written informational materials related to care of the sick were not available for self-education. During this period of time in American nursing, nurses were not educated in any formal sense (Donahue, 1996; Kalisch & Kalisch, 2004).

Advances in Practice

UP UNTIL THE MID-1700s, THERE were no hospitals in what is now the United States. The colonies instead had almshouses where poverty-stricken homeless people were sent if they were sick. Most of the major cities also erected pesthouses, which were makeshift hospitals for contagious diseases. These pesthouses were used for the purpose of isolating sick people from the community rather than providing treatments or nursing care (Kalisch & Kalisch, 2004). For the most part, outside of whatever assistance family or neighbors could provide based on superstition, tradition, and herb lore, there was little help for ill or injured people in the colonies during this time. Sick, injured, or childbearing people were often subjected to crude forms of treatment such as bleeding and purgatives, which worsened illnesses and other physical conditions rather than support healing (Brinkley, 2003; Ulrich, 1990).

The first hospital in the colonies opened in 1751 in Philadelphia through the efforts of Dr. Thomas Bond and Benjamin Franklin. It was named Pennsylvania Hospital. The second colonial hospital was New York Hospital, opened in 1791. These

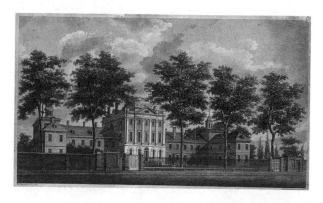

Pennsylvania Hospital, by William Strickland, 1755

were the only two hospitals in the colonies opened before 1800. They were built, organized, and managed much the same as hospitals in Great Britain (Donahue, 1996) and, even though the creation of hospitals might be seen as an advancement in health care, they initially did not offer substantial outcome improvements for patients over and above staying home and attempting to recover with the assistance of family and friends.

In Europe, advancements related to health care during the 1600s and 1700s included William Harvey's 1619 explanation of how blood circulated throughout the human body. Also, between 1632 and 1723, Anton van Leeuwenhoek discovered protozoa, bacteria, and human spermatozoa after improving an existing microscope to magnify objects up to 270 times. These events did not result in significant improvements of prevailing healthcare interventions for colonists, but they paved the way for future progress.

War and Its Effects on Nursing

THE REVOLUTIONARY WAR, WHICH BEGAN in 1775 and ended with the surrender of the British at Yorktown in 1781, resulted in the creation of an independent nation, the United States of America. At the start of the war, the Revolutionary army was hastily assembled and ill-prepared for the realities of combat, with no medical corps, no Red Cross, and no trained

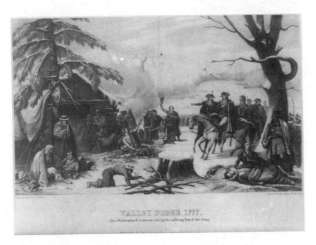

"Valley Forge, 1777—
Gen. Washington and
Lafayette visiting the
suffering Part of the
Army"

nurses (Donahue, 1996). In 1777, George Washington ordered that women be brought in to the military camps to provide nursing care to the soldiers, and many women were subsequently hired and paid two dollars a month for their services. These hired nurses ended up doing more cooking and cleaning than nursing (Donahue, 1996). Laywomen and self-proclaimed nurses were also involved. During the 7 years of war that touched lives and regions in nearly every colony, many women, referred to as camp followers, accompanied their relatives to the front lines and, in addition to cooking, cleaning and mending, assumed unpaid, unofficial nursing roles for the ill and injured (Brinkley, 2003; Collins, 2003).

The efforts of all of the untrained (official and unofficial) nurses during the Revolutionary War did not result in significant advances in nursing immediately following the war. After the fighting ended and the soldiers were released from duty, these women returned home to familiar roles related to hearth and family.

Nursing Workforce Issues

ONE NURSING WORKFORCE ISSUE ALLUDED to in the Image of Nursing section of this chapter will be revisited here. It is a situation that started in Great Britain and continued in the colonies. For the first time in recorded history, the idea of men in nursing became socially unacceptable.

In Great Britain and Europe before the Reformation, nursing work was considered to be appropriate for both men and women. Monks (men) in Catholic religious orders frequently cared for the sick (Donahue, 1996; Kalisch & Kalisch, 2004). Men outside of religious orders also engaged in nursing activities; for example, in military nursing orders, knights were expected to care for the sick and injured when not engaged in battle. These military orders lasted during wartime and then were discontinued, offering no lasting situations where men regularly engaged in nursing care (Donahue, 1996; Kalisch & Kalisch, 2004). The Reformation and the Thirty Years' War resulted in the destruction, closure, or disbanding of many all-male monasteries that provided care for the sick. The Catholic Church shifted responsibility for this activity to nuns (women) and the concept of men in nursing was no longer widely accepted. This sentiment would not begin to change for hundreds of years (Donahue, 1996; Kalisch & Kalisch, 2004).

Licensure and Regulation

NURSES IN THE AMERICAN COLONIES during the 1600s and 1700s were not licensed or formally regulated in any way (Donahue, 1996; Kalisch & Kalisch, 2004).

Nursing Research

RESEARCH RELATED TO NURSING WAS not evident during the 1600s and 1700s.

Summary

NURSING IN THE AMERICAN COLONIES during the 1600s and 1700s was not organized or standardized in any way. The word *nurse* conjured up images of incompetent and unsavory laywomen, a remnant of public perceptions created in Europe and Great Britain. It was not acceptable for men to engage in nursing care. Religious orders of nuns devoted to the care of the sick had not yet been established in the colonies. There were two hospitals in the entire region with poorly trained physicians and untrained nurses where healthcare practices were not particularly supportive of recovery (Donahue, 1996). Women with a desire to earn extra income by helping neighbors who were ill, injured, or in childbirth could assume the role of nurse unfettered by the need for education, licensure, or regulation. The participation of official and unofficial (though all untrained) nurses in care of soldiers during the Revolutionary War did not consequentially alter the state of nursing in America. The stage was set for change.

⬥ IDEAS FOR FURTHER EXPLORATION

1. Explore the history of the nation's first hospital, Pennsylvania Hospital (http://www.uphs.upenn.edu/paharc/). This hospital, which was founded by Benjamin Franklin and Dr. Thomas Bond in 1751, is still serving the people of Philadelphia today.
2. Research medicinal herbs that were used to treat the sick and injured in early American history.
3. Learn more about military nursing orders in Europe. Search for information about Knights Hospitalers of St. Lazarus, Knights of Malta, Knights Templar, Knights of Rhodes, and Knights of St. John of Jerusalem.
4. Research the many roles of women during the Revolutionary War.

❖ DISCUSSION QUESTIONS: APPLICATION TO CURRENT PRACTICE

1. Consider current popular portrayals of nurses as sexually available vixens or frighteningly dour matrons. Either (or both) of these images can be seen in lingerie and Halloween costumes, novelty items, on television, and in the movies. Do you think that the image of nurses in Great Britain that started in the late 1500s and was perpetuated during colonial times and onward has anything to do with this persistent image of nurses at the present time? Explain your answer.

2. How do current media images of nursing affect nurses in particular and the nursing profession in general? Should nurses attempt to change popular perceptions? Why or why not?

3. Colonists used a variety of folk remedies and herbs to treat illnesses and injury. Many early healthcare interventions might seem ridiculous to today's nurses who cannot envision using these types of treatments in modern health care. Surprisingly, many antiquated treatments are receiving a second look in today's healthcare arena—for example, leeches. Leeches have been used by many cultures for various healthcare concerns for centuries, and they were used during the American colonial period to treat a variety of ailments. They later fell out of use in favor of more modern interventions. Current nurses are again using leeches for management of wounds and limb reattachments. Can you think of any other folk or herbal remedies from the past that are reemerging as important healthcare treatment alternatives?

⩗ MeSH SEARCH TERMS

Nursing can be used as a subject heading combined with one of the terms listed here or as a subheading (Revolutionary War/nursing). When searching the Web, use quotation marks around phrases where you want your search terms to appear right next to each other (such as "Dorothea Dix"). These medical subject heading (MeSH) terms can be used to search medical literature databases like Medline/PubMed:

Almshouses   Hospitals, religious
American Revolution   Nursing

⩗ SUGGESTED READING

Barry, J. & Jones, C. (1994). *Medicine and charity before the welfare state.* London: Routledge.

Larrabee, E. (1971). *The benevolent and necessary institution: The New York Hospital, 1771–1971.* Garden City, NY: Doubleday.

Wilbur, C. K. (1997). *Revolutionary medicine, 1700–1800.* Philadelphia: Chelsea House.

Williams, W. H. (1976). *America's first hospital: The Pennsylvania Hospital, 1751–1841.* Wayne, PA: Haverford House.

⊕ REFERENCES

Brinkley, A. (2003). *American history: A survey.* New York: McGraw-Hill.

Collins, G. (2003). *America's women: 400 years of dolls, drudges, helpmates, and heroines.* New York: William Morrow.

Donahue, M. P. (1996). *Nursing: The finest art* (2nd ed.). St. Louis, MO: Mosby.

Kalisch, P. A. & Kalisch, B. J. (2004). *American nursing: A history* (4th ed.). Philadelphia: Lippincott, Williams, & Wilkins.

Ulrich, L. T. (1990). *A midwife's tale: The life of Martha Ballard based on her diary, 1785–1812.* New York: Knopf, distributed by Random House.

Prelude to Modern American Nursing

1845
Nightingale announces she wants to be a nurse; meets familial and societal resistance

1837
Nightingale believes she is 'called to serve'

| 1800 | 1805 | 1810 | 1815 | 1820 | 1825 | 1830 | 1835 | 1840 | 1845 |

1820
Florence Nightingale born in Florence, Italy to a wealthy, upper-class family

1837–1850 Nightingale notices social conditions and writes about them

THE WORK OF FLORENCE NIGHTINGALE

Kathleen Sitzman

1850–1851 Nightingale trains in nursing in Kaiserwerth, Germany

1854–1856 Nightingale revolutionizes nursing care in hospitals during Crimean War

1854–1897 Nightingale writes many letters on nursing

1910 Nightingale dies in London

1850　1855　1860　1865　1870　1875　1880　1885　1890　1895　1900

1854
Nightingale and other nurses are stationed at the Barrack Hospital in Scutari, Turkey

1858
Nightingale becomes first female member of the Statistical Society of London

1860
• Nightingale publishes *Notes on Nursing*
• Nightingale opens a nurse training school at St. Thomas' Hospital in London

1869
Nightingale and Dr. Elizabeth Blackwell open the Women's Medical College

OUR NURSING HERITAGE: KEY PEOPLE

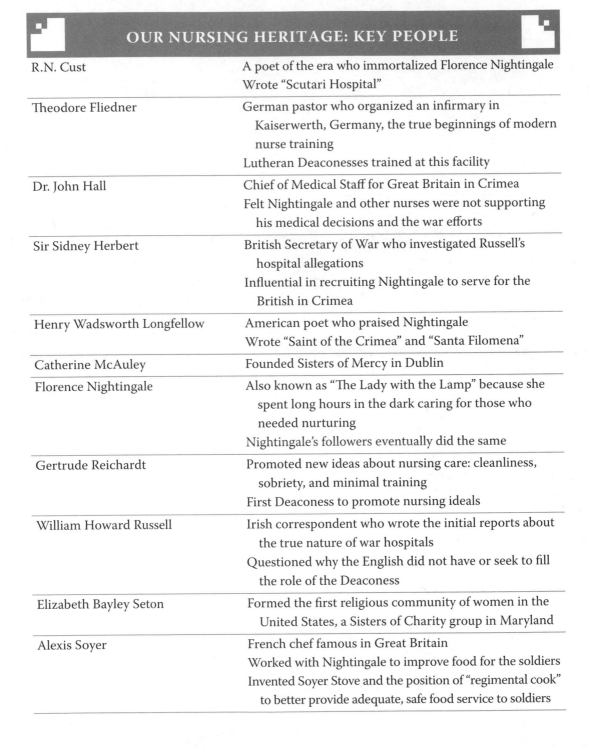

R.N. Cust	A poet of the era who immortalized Florence Nightingale Wrote "Scutari Hospital"
Theodore Fliedner	German pastor who organized an infirmary in Kaiserwerth, Germany, the true beginnings of modern nurse training Lutheran Deaconesses trained at this facility
Dr. John Hall	Chief of Medical Staff for Great Britain in Crimea Felt Nightingale and other nurses were not supporting his medical decisions and the war efforts
Sir Sidney Herbert	British Secretary of War who investigated Russell's hospital allegations Influential in recruiting Nightingale to serve for the British in Crimea
Henry Wadsworth Longfellow	American poet who praised Nightingale Wrote "Saint of the Crimea" and "Santa Filomena"
Catherine McAuley	Founded Sisters of Mercy in Dublin
Florence Nightingale	Also known as "The Lady with the Lamp" because she spent long hours in the dark caring for those who needed nurturing Nightingale's followers eventually did the same
Gertrude Reichardt	Promoted new ideas about nursing care: cleanliness, sobriety, and minimal training First Deaconess to promote nursing ideals
William Howard Russell	Irish correspondent who wrote the initial reports about the true nature of war hospitals Questioned why the English did not have or seek to fill the role of the Deaconess
Elizabeth Bayley Seton	Formed the first religious community of women in the United States, a Sisters of Charity group in Maryland
Alexis Soyer	French chef famous in Great Britain Worked with Nightingale to improve food for the soldiers Invented Soyer Stove and the position of "regimental cook" to better provide adequate, safe food service to soldiers

Grey Sisters, Daughters of Charity, Sisters of St. Vincent de Paul, and other female orders of nursing in the United States	Females took simple vows to care for the sick and the needy
Nightingale's Nurses	Assisted with hospital reform and interventions Willing to change status quo

Sociopolitical Climate

THROUGHOUT HER LIFE, FLORENCE NIGHTINGALE effected great social and political change while, for the most part, working within the sociopolitical constraints of her time where women were not allowed to inhabit leadership roles. Women were expected to be homemakers if that were financially feasible, or if necessary, to work outside the home in menial jobs that did not provide opportunities for power or influence. While Nightingale eschewed homemaking in favor of becoming a nurse and then pursuing widespread public policy changes that would improve health care, she still avoided assuming roles that were considered inappropriate for women.

> She did not accept overt leadership positions, but worked behind the scenes, allowing those who worked with her to take credit....Women, with the exception of the Queen of England, were not allowed to speak at Parliament. To influence her causes, Nightingale had to utilize "referent power," working with others in private and through others' public offices and external influence. (Andrist, Nicholas, & Wolf, 2006, p. 478)

Although she lived and worked in Great Britain, Nightingale significantly influenced the evolution of modern nursing in the United States. Her revolutionary approaches related to nursing, military healthcare reform, sanitation, nursing education, and the organization of hospitals transformed health care in Europe and the United States during her lifetime and up to the present day.

A Child of Privilege Chooses a Life of Service

Florence Nightingale was born on May 12, 1820 in Florence, Italy, to affluent British parents during an extended honeymoon trip that lasted over 3 years. Her only sibling, a sister named Parthenope, had been born a year earlier

(Dossey, 2000). Nightingale grew up in England, shuttling between country and city estates in concurrence with the London social seasons. She received a thorough education under the direction of her father, William Edward Nightingale, who was a Cambridge scholar. Social norms of the day dictated that upper class women should marry well and focus on family and social matters. Nightingale's mother, Frances (Fanny), was a conventional woman who strictly followed social norms and wanted her daughters to do the same.

Nightingale preferred to focus on developing her intellect, earnestly studying with her father and various nannies. She was a prolific letter writer by the age of 7 and wrote an autobiography entirely in French between the ages of 8 and 10. She could speak seven languages and had special talent in writing and mathematics. She was also devoted to service work and, from an early age, often cared for ill family members, servants, and neighbors (Dossey, 2000; MacQueen, 2007). Upon reaching her teen years, she increased her service-related activities by providing funded medical care, food, and fabric (for the purpose of sewing clothing) to economically disadvantaged neighbors (Dossey, 2000; MacQueen, 2007).

As the Nightingale daughters grew into adulthood, Parthenope increasingly engaged in homemaking, entertaining, and social networking; however, Florence's resistance to participation in such things, coupled with her refusal to marry, caused great consternation for her family. Furthermore, Florence's fervent interest in nursing was judged to be odd and highly inappropriate, and Florence's mother repeatedly forbade Florence from pursuing a life devoted to nursing (Dossey, 2000). Nightingale persevered against vigorous objections from her family and in 1851, at the age of 31, went to study nursing in Germany at the deaconess training center at Kaiserswerth. She returned home and eventually worked as the head of the Institute for the Care of Sick Gentlewomen on Harley Street in London until the outbreak of the Crimean War resulted in circumstances that would change her life (Donahue, 1996; Kalisch & Kalisch, 2004).

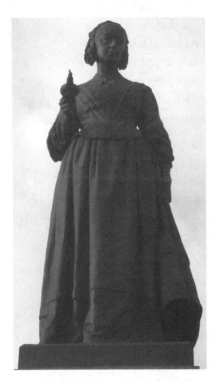

Florence Nightingale Monument in London, England

The Image of Nursing

THE PERIOD OF TIME FROM the 1840s through the 1860s, when Nightingale would have been in her 20s, 30s, and 40s, is often referred to as a dark period in nursing (Donahue, 1996; Kalisch & Kalisch, 2004) because nursing conditions were at their worst and general public perception of nursing was at its lowest. The forced closing of monastery hospitals during the Reformation, coupled with a proliferation of poorly staffed and managed public hospitals where nurses were culled from the lowest dregs of society, had resulted in a deplorable situation in relation to professional nursing. Many writers and political cartoonists in Great Britain during the mid-1800s and early 1900s immortalized the unfavorable public perception of nursing in editorial cartoons and prose. Charles Dickens, a celebrated novelist during this time whose work was widely read by the literate population, created the despicable characters of Sairy Gamp (private duty nurse) and Betsy Prig (hospital nurse) in his highly popular novel *Martin Chuzzlewit,* published in 1844. Dickens's introductory description of Sairy Gamp in Chapter 19 of *Martin Chuzzlewit* presented an unsavory character who smelled of alcohol, had snuff all over her shabby dress, manipulated clients into providing her with new clothing, and equally savored attending a birth or a death:

> She was a fat old woman, this Mrs. Gamp, with a husky voice and a moist eye, which she had a remarkable power of turning up, and only showing the white of it. Having very little neck, it cost her some trouble to look over herself, if one may say so, at those to whom she talked. She wore a very rusty black gown, rather the worse for snuff, and a shawl and bonnet to correspond. In these dilapidated articles of dress she had, on principle, arrayed herself, time out of mind, on such occasions as the present; for this at once expressed a decent amount of veneration for the deceased, and invited the next of kin to present her with a fresher suit of weeds: an appeal so frequently successful, that the very fetch and ghost of Mrs. Gamp, bonnet and all, might be seen hanging up, any hour in the day, in at least a dozen of the second-hand clothes shops about Holborn. The face of Mrs. Gamp— the nose in particular—was somewhat red and swollen, and it was difficult to enjoy her society without becoming conscious of a smell of spirits. Like most persons who have attained to great eminence in their profession, she

took to hers very kindly; insomuch that, setting aside her natural predilec-
tions as a woman, she went to a lying-in or a laying-out with equal zest and
relish. (Dickens, 1844, pp. 291–292)

Sairy Gamp and Betsy Prig were the best known literary images that
illustrated public perception of nurses during Nightingale's adult life. Nurses
during this dark period were viewed as:

> ... illiterate, rough, inconsiderate, oftentimes immoral or alcoholic. When
> a woman could no longer earn a living from gambling or vice, she might
> become a nurse. Nurses were drawn from among discharged patients, pris-
> oners, and the lowest strata of society.... There was little organization
> associated with nursing and certainly no social standing. (Dossey, 2000,
> p. 191)

Nightingale was fully aware of the poor reputation of nurses and sought
to change the image of nursing. She cultivated working relationships with
journalists, philanthropists, lawmakers, and administrators and lobbied to
improve overall conditions for nurses so that patient care would improve
and respectable women would be drawn to the profession. Nightingale outlined standards related to personal comportment and decorum for nurses
that included directives for morality, self-restraint, and devotion to service.
She asserted that spirituality had a place in nursing and that nursing should
be considered a calling rather than simply a job (Dossey, 1996). Her views
on nursing, published in newspapers, magazine articles, and in her best-
selling book, *Notes on Nursing* (1860), strongly influenced the vision of professional nursing that immigrated to the United States from the mid-19th
century onward (Andrist et al., 2006). Nightingale's work essentially marked
the beginning of the end of the dark period of nursing.

The Education of Nurses

AFTER RETURNING FROM THE CRIMEAN WAR (which is discussed in
greater detail in the War and Its Effects on Nursing section of this
chapter), Nightingale was considered the foremost authority on nursing
in Great Britain, Europe, and the United States by the general public, and
she sought to use this notoriety for the betterment of nursing. Nightingale
believed that organized nursing education would provide a means to raise

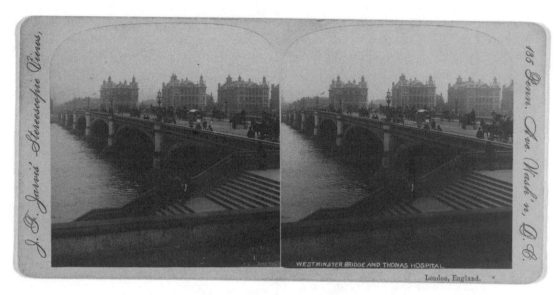

"Westminster Bridge and Thomas Hospital," London, England

nursing to a respectable endeavor by clarifying standards for professional and personal conduct and standardizing how nurses provided care for the sick. Against the objections of physicians in England but with the support of a charitable foundation (the Nightingale Fund) and numerous colleagues, Nightingale opened a nurse training school at St. Thomas Hospital in London on June 24, 1860 (Dossey, 2000). This was the first school of its kind. The objectives were to train hospital and district (home care) nurses and to teach nurses how to instruct other nurses. There were ordinary nursing students (probationers), drawn from relatively uneducated middle-class ranks, whose expenses were paid by the Nightingale Fund.

> The nurse probationers, who had to sign a 4-year contract, were to be admitted free of charge and were to receive free room and board, their own tea and sugar, a washing allowance, and a wage of 10 Lira for their first year. (Donahue, 1996, p. 222)

Students (probationers) were taught how to provide direct patient care in hospital and home settings for 1 year, after which time they worked as staff nurses at St. Thomas Hospital or another approved hospital for a minimum of 3 years. There were also "Lady Nurse" students, gentlewomen who paid their own expenses and were expected to become future matrons (nursing instructors and supervisors) (Donahue, 1996). The Nightingale Training School served as a model for the establishment of other nursing schools across England, Europe, and the United States. The Nightingale Training School's training model, coupled with the visibility of nurse graduates who were highly sought after in England and elsewhere, helped open up a new and respectable career option for women all over the world.

In addition to establishing the first nurse training school and providing a model for other schools to emulate, Nightingale published a 79-page book meant to explain how to provide effective nursing care in the home, entitled *Notes on Nursing* (1860), which became a best seller. Although this text was aimed at helping laywomen understand how to provide basic nursing care to family members, it was used as a nursing text at the Nightingale Training School and is now recognized as the earliest modern nursing text (Dossey, 2000; Kalisch & Kalisch, 2004).

Advances in Practice

I N *NOTES ON NURSING* (1860), Nightingale introduced her then unheard-of revolutionary ideas related to holistic nursing care that are now familiar to any modern nurse.

> In watching diseases, both in private houses and in public hospitals, the thing which strikes the experienced observer most forcibly is this, that the symptoms or the sufferings generally considered to be inevitable and incident to the disease are very often not symptoms of the disease at all, but of something quite different—of the want of fresh air, or of light, or of warmth, or of quiet, or of cleanliness, or of punctuality and care in the administration of diet, of each or of all of these ... I use the word nursing for want of a better. It has been limited to signify little more than the administration of medicines and the application of poultices. It ought to signify the proper use of fresh air, light, warmth, cleanliness, quiet, and the proper selection and administration of diet—all at the least expense of vital power to the patient. (Nightingale, 1860, p. 8)

It was not yet understood that germs or filth could cause or worsen illness and/or infection, and the value of simple cleanliness in relation to well-being was not yet embraced by healthcare providers of the time, but Nightingale had observed through many years of experience that patients fared better in clean, light, calm, well-ventilated surroundings. Nightingale believed that it was imperative to fully attend to a patient's total environment in order to provide support for the body's own healing powers to resolve illness (Nightingale, 1860). Although these concepts may seem to be commonplace and common sense today, in Nightingale's time, they represented great advancement in nursing practice and in health care. This approach was the beginning of a holistic patient care model that persists to this day.

In addition to creating a holistic approach to patient care, Nightingale was the first nurse to systematically collect data and then statistically analyze it in order to justify proposed policy and treatment protocol changes aimed at improving patient outcomes (Andrist et al., 2006). This activity was a precursor to the current evidence-based practice movement. It is interesting to note that in 1858, because of her extensive understanding of and use of statistics, Nightingale became the first female member of the Statistical Society of London (Dossey, 2000). Based on her study and statistical analysis of information related to hospital surgical data, the sanitary situation in hospitals in India, Crimean War mortalities, and the British army medical department, Nightingale made many fruitful recommendations for change to improve patient outcomes in Great Britain and India. Nightingale also systematically collected and documented health and illness data from public census records, believing that such information could provide the basis for sweeping improvement of public health (Dossey, 2000). Throughout her life, she used her knowledge and expertise related to statistical analysis to support productive collaborations with members of the English Parliament, political reformers, philanthropists, and journalists.

War and Its Effects on Nursing

IN 1853, THE TURKS WERE engaged in a war with Russia on Turkish soil—the Crimean War. In 1854, in an attempt to end the war and stabilize the region, France and Britain demanded that Russia withdraw from Turkey. When Russia refused, France and Britain sent troops to Turkey to aid in the expulsion of the Russians. There was great bloodshed among British soldiers. British military hospitals in Turkey were ill-equipped and poorly managed, resulting in unnecessary suffering and death among British soldiers. A war correspondent for the London *Times*, William Howard Russell, exposed the seriously substandard military hospital situation in Turkey, which inflamed British public opinion (Dossey, 2000). Amid great public outcry and vigorous demands for improved care of wounded British soldiers in the Crimea, British Secretary at War Sidney Herbert took the unprecedented step of making plans to send a contingent of female nurses to the Barrack Hospital at Scutari in an attempt to improve conditions. He asked 34-year-old Florence Nightingale to lead the expedition (Dossey, 2000). On October 21, 1854, Nightingale, whom Herbert had just appointed superintendent of the female nursing establishment of the English general hospitals in Turkey, and 38 nurses departed London for the Barrack Hospital at Scutari (Donahue, 1996). The conditions that awaited this determined and brave group of women were far worse than any of them imagined. The huge Barrack Hospital, which was designed to hold 1,700 patients, had been filled with between 3,000 and 4,000 wounded and dying soldiers. There were few windows in the cavernous stone building, and candles stuck in empty beer bottles illuminated row upon row (4 miles of rows in one estimate) of filthy, blood-covered, suffering, dying, emaciated men without blankets, sheets, or the most basic hygiene necessities, lying in their own excrement. Lice, maggots, various other vermin, and rats were everywhere and crawled over the wounded soldiers. There was a lack of even the most basic medical supplies, no kitchen facilities, and no laundry facilities. The mortality rate was 60 percent (Donahue, 1996; Kalisch & Kalisch, 2004). The military physicians and officers resented the presence of female nurses and were unhelpful and abusive. Accommodations for the nurses consisted of six tiny, squalid rooms with no furniture. The nurses received one meager meal a day (Donahue, 1996; Kalisch & Kalisch, 2004). Nevertheless, Nightingale used her considerable influence back home to obtain needed supplies and more nurses. She worked tirelessly day and night to transform the Barrack Hospital at Scutari into a place of healing. War correspondents and recovering soldiers sent messages to Britain praising the work of Nightingale and her contingent of nurses. London *Times* Correspondent M. W. MacDonald filed this report on November 20, 1854:

Wherever there is disease in its most dangerous form, and the hand of the despoiler distressingly nigh, there is this incomparable woman [Florence Nightingale] sure to be seen; her benignant presence is an influence for good comfort, even amid the struggles of expiring nature. She is a "ministering angel," without any exaggeration, in these hospitals; her slender form glides quietly along each corridor, every poor fellow's face softens with gratitude at the sight of her. When all of the medical officers have retired for the night, and silence and darkness have settled down upon those miles of prostrate sick, she may be observed alone, with a little lamp in her hand, making her solitary rounds. (Kalisch & Kalisch, 2004, p. 32)

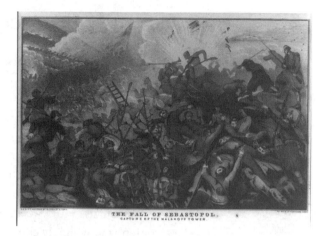

"The Fall of Sebastopol, Capture of the Malakoff Tower," 1854–1855

Nightingale worked to exhaustion and near collapse. She contracted Crimean fever and almost died. Her efforts at the Barrack Hospital in Scutari resulted in the mortality rate decreasing from 60 percent to a fraction over 1 percent. She returned to England a national hero after the war ended in 1856. The extreme hardship Nightingale endured during the Crimean War resulted in frail health for the rest of her life (Donahue, 1996; Dossey, 2000; Kalisch & Kalisch, 2004).

Nightingale's experiences in the Crimea impassioned her to work for healthcare reform for British soldiers. She labored ceaselessly and successfully (due to her immense popularity, expertise, experience, and collegial connections) to improve military hospital conditions. She also worked to improve civilian hospitals and health care. As a result of the great public stature of Nightingale following the Crimean War, a philanthropic organization named the Nightingale Fund was set up by colleagues and supporters to aid Nightingale in her work. Money from this fund was used in the establishment of the Nightingale Training School at St. Thomas Hospital in London and later for other nurse training schools in England.

Nursing Workforce Issues

Nursing workforce issues during nightingale's life were related to the conscription of women in questionable circumstances into nursing work because there was a severe shortage of willing respectable women to work as nurses. Nightingale did much to address this issue. She created widely accepted guidelines and standards for professional comportment, education, and patient care. The Nightingale vision of nursing became entrenched by the late 1800s, making nursing a respectable occupational endeavor for women. As a result of Nightingale's reforms, the nursing workforce stabilized into a relatively homogenous group of single middle-class women who willingly chose to be nurses. It is important to note that Nightingale did not support the idea of men in nursing, feeling that it was an exclusively female occupation, so men were essentially excluded from nursing during this time (Evans, 2004).

Licensure and Regulation

Nurses during nightingale's time were not licensed or formally regulated (Donahue, 1996; Kalisch & Kalisch, 2004); however, names of the graduates of the Nightingale Training School were entered into a school register as certificated (Dossey, 2000, p. 302). Other nurse training schools kept similar registers, but there was no coordinated or organized effort between schools, cities, regions, or countries. Quality of training and level of skill among graduates from different schools was not uniform (Kalisch & Kalisch, 2004).

Nursing Research

Nightingale engaged in a method of inquiry that could be described today as retrospective study. Retrospective studies are those in which a researcher or group of researchers studies and analyzes events that have occurred in the past in order to find relationships between documented phenomena (Polit and Beck, 2008). Nightingale engaged in this type of inquiry continually throughout her lifetime, for example by studying hospital records to discover relationships between hospital mortality and specific treatments in order to discern what treatments worked best for certain conditions (Dossey, 1996). Nightingale used her findings to justify proposed treatment protocol and healthcare policy changes. Other than Nightingale's undertakings, there is no record of any concerted effort among other nurses of her time to engage in research.

Summary

F LORENCE NIGHTINGALE WAS A BRILLIANT, visionary, driven woman. She became a nurse despite great resistance from those closest to her at a time when nursing was at its lowest point in history. She envisioned what nursing *could* be and then set about bringing this vision to fruition. Her entire life was devoted to the betterment of nursing and health care. She created a model of nursing that persists to this day in the form of honor and respectability associated with nurses, highly structured nursing education, and holistic patient care approaches. She was ahead of her time, engaging in research and effecting sweeping policy changes when women were heavily discouraged from such endeavors. Nightingale's legacy is evident in nursing worldwide and will continue to influence the profession into the future.

⚬ IDEAS FOR FURTHER EXPLORATION

1. Learn more about Great Britain's involvement in the Crimean War to better understand the obstacles that Nightingale faced during her work in the Barrack Hospital at Scutari.
2. Find and read a research study with a retrospective study design to gain a deeper appreciation for the type of research in which Nightingale engaged.
3. Research the evidence-based practice movement in nursing in the United States and compare your findings to Nightingale's early work.
4. Florence Nightingale's work was extensive and involved many areas not covered in this chapter. To learn more about this remarkable nurse leader, read: Dossey, B. M. (2000). *Florence Nightingale: Mystic, visionary, healer.* Pennsylvania: Springhouse.

⚜ DISCUSSION QUESTIONS: APPLICATION TO CURRENT PRACTICE

1. Nightingale's work is still evident in current nursing education and practice. What do you believe is Florence Nightingale's greatest contribution to modern nursing? Explain your answer using examples from your own clinical experiences.

2. Do you believe that there are aspects of Nightingale's work that hindered the professional development of nursing? Explain your answer using examples from your own clinical experiences.

3. There are many preconceptions about Florence Nightingale among nurses and laypeople. Compare your preconceived notions about Nightingale to what you learned in this chapter. What was the most surprising thing you learned?

4. Nightingale was heavily involved in politics throughout her life as she labored to improve nursing and health care. She believed that professional nurses should become politically involved when necessary to effect change related to health care-related issues. Identify one healthcare-related issue that affects your current nursing practice and present a plan for your participation in the political process to effect change.

⚜ MeSH SEARCH TERMS

Florence Nightingale does not have her own MeSH term in Medline/PubMed. When searching the Web for information on Nightingale, try searching her name as a phrase in quotation marks: "Florence Nightingale." Phrase searching would also be beneficial when searching for Nightingale's work "Notes on Nursing" and the "Nightingale School of Nursing."

⚜ SUGGESTED READING

Dossey, B. M. (2000). *Florence Nightingale: Mystic, visionary, healer.* Springhouse, PA: Springhouse.

Gill, G. (2004). *Nightingales: The extraordinary upbringing and curious life of Miss Florence Nightingale.* New York: Ballantine.

Hobbs, C. A. (1997). *Florence Nightingale.* New York: Prentice-Hall International.

Nightingale, F. (1860). *Notes on nursing: What it is and what it is not.* New York: D. Appleton & Company.

Smith, F. B. (1982). *Florence Nightingale: Reputation and power.* New York: St. Martin's Press.

Vicinus, M., & Nergaard, B. (1990). *Ever yours, Florence Nightingale: Selected letters.* Cambridge, MA: Harvard University Press.

◆ REFERENCES

Andrist, L. C., Nicholas, P. K., & Wolf, K. A. (Eds.). (2006). *A history of nursing ideas.* Sudbury, MA: Jones and Bartlett.

Dickens, C. (1844). *Martin Chuzzlewit.* New York: Dodd, Mead, and Co.

Donahue, M. P. (1996). *Nursing: The finest art.* Philadelphia: Mosby.

Dossey, B. M. (2000). *Florence Nightingale: Mystic, visionary, healer.* Springhouse, PA: Springhouse.

Evans, J. (2004). Men nurses: A historical and feminist perspective. *Journal of Advanced Nursing, 47*(3), 321–328.

Kalisch, P. A. & Kalisch, B. J. (2004). *American nursing: A history* (4th ed.). Philadelphia: Lippincott, Williams, & Wilkins.

MacQueen, J. S. (2007). Florence Nightingale's nursing practice. *Nursing History Review, 15,* 29–49.

Nightingale, F. (1860). *Notes on nursing: What it is and what it is not.* New York: D. Appleton & Company.

Polit, D. F. and Beck, C. T. (2008). *Nursing research: Generating and assessing evidence for nursing practice.* Philadelphia: Wolters Kluwer Health/Lippincott, Williams, and Wilkins.

CHAPTER 4

Nursing in the United States During the 1800s

1790–1817 Three hospitals for the chronically mentally ill are created

1800–1850 Whiskey or brandy used for pain management and anesthesia

1800–1880 Most nurses are untrained

1800–1900 Country doctors are common

1812–1815 War of 1812

1817–1898 Indian Wars

1830–1850 Nursing school in Kaiserwerth, Germany sparks the nursing education movement

1800	1805	1810	1815	1820	1825	1830	1835	1840	1845

1844
Sairy Gamp, nurse and midwife, appears in Charles Dickens' *Martin Chuzzlewit*
1846
Ether used for anesthesia

1840–1865 Dorothea Dix promotes mental health

1840–1900 Early understanding of sanitation and asepsis develops from work of Pasteur, Lister, Koch, Halsted, Virchow, and others

1846–1848 Mexican War

INSPIRATION AND INSIGHT LEAD TO NURSING REFORMS

Kathleen Sitzman

1861–1865 U.S. Civil War
- Dix organizes care for soldiers in the North
- Kate Cumming organizes female nurses in the South

1870–1900 Medical and surgical advancements in special procedures and equipment (i.e. X-ray, stethoscope)

1850	1855	1860	1865	1870	1875	1880	1885	1890	1895	1900

1850
Health Almanac sold to the public; contains "secret" health formulas

1854–1956 Crimean War prompts work of Florence Nightingale

1862
New England Hospital for Women and Children opens; has its own nurse training program

1868
American Medical Association (AMA) advocates for training for nurses

1873
Nursing schools opened in Boston, MA, New York, NY, and New Haven, CT

1877
Sister Mary Bernard is the first nurse anesthesia specialist

1879
- First Black nursing student graduates (Mary Mahoney)
- First all-Black nursing school opened at Spelman Seminary in Atlanta, GA

1880
Ether and chloroform used for anesthesia

1886–1898 Five schools for male nurses open

1898–1902 Spanish–American War

OUR NURSING HERITAGE: KEY PEOPLE

Louisa May Alcott	Volunteered as a nurse in the Civil War
	Wrote *Hospital Sketches*—A humorous work based on her experiences
Elizabeth Blackwell	First woman in the U.S. to study medicine officially and receive her M.D. degree
	Collaborated with Lillian Wald and Mary Brewster
	Established a nursing school at Bellevue Hospital
	Established the New York Infirmary for Women and Children
Mary Brewster	Offered care to the needy in tenements
	Worked with Lillian Wald
	Helped organize nursing in the community
'Mother' Mary Ann Bickerdyke	Untrained nurse who worked for the Union Army in the Civil War
	Superb provision of care earned her the title of 'Mother'
Kate Cumming	Volunteer Confederate nurse
	Kept a journal of her experiences that described nursing in the South
Hattie P. Dame	Civil War Nurse who encouraged total patient care
	President of the Army Nurses Association
Dorothea Lynde Dix	Crusaded for reform of treatment for the mentally ill
	Superintendent of Army Nurses in the Civil War
René Laennec	Invented the stethoscope
Clara Maass	Spanish American War nurse
	Died in her efforts as a human subject for Yellow Fever research
Mary P. Mahoney	First professional Black nurse
	Co-founder of the National Association of Colored Graduate Nurses
	Completed one of the first accelerated nurse training programs

Linda Richards	America's first officially trained nurse
	First Superintendent of Nurses at Massachusetts General Hospital
Isabel Hampton Robb	First president of the American Nurses Association
	Organized the Nurses' Associated Alumnae of the United States and Canada
Wilhelm Konrad Roentgen	Invented the X-ray
Lillian Wald	Established the Henry Street Settlement
	Credited with the idea of visiting nurse services and public and school nursing
Walt Whitman	Male nurse for the Union Army in the Civil War
	Author and poet who wrote about hospital care, in addition to other works
Jane Stuart Woolsey	Nurse recruited to work in Union hospitals
	Attempted to bring order to care despite untrained nurses
	Defined what a nurse was at that time in *Hospital Days*
Marie Zakrzewska	One of the first female physicians in the United States
	Promoted care of women and children
Oliver Wendell Holmes	All made contributions and discoveries about asepsis and bateriology
Robert Koch	
Joseph Lister	
Louis Pasteur	
Robert Virchow	

Sociopolitical Climate

DUE TO COMMON LAW AND biblical tradition, American women in the 1800s were considered inferior in strength and intellect and superior in terms of morality. Men were expected to protect women and provide guidance, structure, and material support. These rigid gender roles may have provided predictability and comfort during the turbulent and rapidly changing times (Brinkley, 2003; Collins, 2003).

The Revolutionary War had ended in 1783, and a postwar depression ensued in 1784, making the economy unstable for a number of years. Just when economic conditions seemed to be improving, the country was again plunged into an economic depression in 1808 (Brinkley, 2003). To add to the tumult, the United States engaged in five wars during the 1800s—the War of 1812 from 1812 to 1815, wherein the British stormed what is now Washington, District of Columbia, and set fire to the White House (Brinkley, 2003); the Indian Wars from 1817 to 1898; the Mexican War from 1846 to 1848; the Civil War from 1861 to 1865; and the Spanish-American War from 1898 to 1902 (United States Department of Veteran's Affairs, 2007). Involvement in five wars contributed to the sociopolitical instability that began with Colonial settlement. Many other issues contributed to instability, including the following:

- In the period of time between the War of 1812 and the start of the Civil War in 1861, the American population grew tremendously, and although the bulk of the population resided in agricultural communities, cities became teeming centers of trade, industry, diversity, and culture (Brinkley, 2003).

- Desire for new farmland and improved economic opportunities prompted Americans to move from populated areas to unexplored regions. Westward migration gained momentum in the 1850s and accelerated throughout the rest of the century, with over 2 million settlers migrating west between 1870 and 1900 (Brinkley, 2003). Clashes between migrating settlers who wanted to partition and own the land and Native Americans who did not agree with the notion of personal ownership of the land resulted in the Indian Wars (Brinkley, 2003).

- The Northern and Southern regions of the United States became increasingly divided over multiple issues such as national policy related to the unsettled western territories and whether or not slavery should be allowed or abolished. Continued contention between the North and South resulted in the Civil War, which lasted from 1861 to 1865 (Brinkley, 2003; Kalisch & Kalisch, 2004).

- The reconstruction period following the Civil War proved challenging as Americans attempted to rebuild the scarred nation amidst economic difficulty and continued animosity between the North and South (Brinkley, 2003).

By the late 1800s, the chaos of war, the privation of economic depression, the hardships associated with the westward migration, and workforce demands created by the industrial revolution resulted in an environment where women had opportunities to work in a variety of nontraditional occupations, for example as factory workers in the industrialized cities and small business operators in the western territories. "Small communities of single working women became common in industrialized nineteenth-century America. Women's newly found passion for work outside the home provided companionships, security, and the means out of the garden...." (Baer, 1989, as cited in D'Antonio, Baer, Rinker, & Lynaugh, 2007, p. 98). Despite new opportunities for women, the majority of nurses (who were overwhelmingly female) remained highly conservative and eschewed female independence in favor of embracing traditional subservient female roles in hospital and private duty settings.

The Image of Nursing

IN THE EARLY 1800S, NURSING work was still considered undesirable for respectable women. The work of Florence Nightingale significantly changed that perception by the mid-1800s, making nursing more acceptable and laudable to the general public, even though earlier negative perceptions lingered in tandem with the newer ones (Donahue, 1996; Kalisch & Kalisch, 2004). In addition to Nightingale's work, the establishment of nurse training schools and the arrival of religious nursing orders in the United States helped to create an image of nursing in the later half of the 1800s of women who were conservative, loyal, docile, submissive, and dedicated to service above personal needs and/or desires.

Nurse uniforms both reflected and influenced the public image of nursing. Before the advent of nurse training schools in the United States, there was no specific type of dress to distinguish nurses from other women, though nurses were advised by Revolutionary War and Civil War matrons to avoid jewelry, fanciness, and hoop skirts and to dress plainly in black, grey, or brown woolen dresses that were modest in design. Hair was to be secured in a bun with a cap over it (Houweling, 2004; Kalisch & Kalisch, 2004). Nurse training schools, where distinctive uniforms were created for probationers and graduate nurses, helped to standardize nursing uniforms for the first time in the United States (Houweling, 2004). The training school uniforms reflected styles of the day, which included full skirts, corsets, and long, billowing sleeves. These styles were bothersome and restrictive in light of typical nursing duties that involved heavy cleaning, cooking, laundering, and direct patient care. Later modifications to improve functionality included detachable sleeves, cuffs, and aprons that allowed for frequent laundering of areas that were regularly soiled. Nurses were expected to keep their uniforms immaculately clean and starched (Houweling, 2004; Kalisch & Kalisch, 2004).

Overall, uniforms associated with nurse training schools that appeared in the mid- to late 1800s were indicative of a changing public image of nursing because they conveyed conservativeness, modesty, dignity, and pride related to the nursing role, in contrast to earlier negative perceptions. The new public image heralded a progression of the nursing profession from the lower echelons of society into a middle-class realm of respectability.

The Education of Nurses

FORMAL NURSING EDUCATION IN AMERICA did not emerge until the later half of the century when, in 1862, Dr. Marie Zakrzewska opened the New England Hospital for Women and Children, which had its own nurse training program. Three more nursing schools, modeled after Nightingale's training school in Great Britain, opened in 1873; one opened at Massachusetts General Hospital in Boston, one at Bellevue Hospital in New York, and one at New Haven Hospital in Connecticut. In 1880, there were 15 nurse training schools in the United States, and by 1900 there were 432 (Andrist, Nicholas, & Wolf, 2006; Hine, 1989). All of these schools were hospital-based and aimed at educating conservative, unmarried, White, middle-class women (Andrist et al., 2006; Kalisch & Kalisch, 2004).

The length of required training for nurses in these early training schools was initially 1 year. Hospital administrators quickly realized that nursing students cheaply provided the bulk of the workforce needed to run a hospital,

including all of the cleaning, food
preparation, laundering, and patient
care. By 1880, the length of required
training increased to 3 years. Probationers (student nurses) typically
began training with heavy cleaning,
cooking, and laundering responsibilities and gradually transitioned to
increased patient care activities as
training progressed. There was strict
discipline, with superintendents over-
seeing every aspect of each proba-
tioner's life, even during time off from
required duties. Obedience in relation to work, dress, habits, and per-

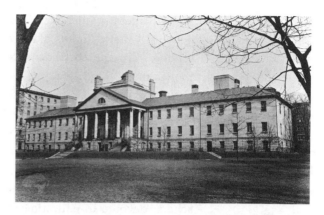

Massachusetts General
Hospital, Bulfinch
Building

sonal behavior was expected at all times. Submission to more experienced
students, superintendents, physicians, and administrators was expected,
and disrespect or misbehavior of any kind provided grounds for dismissal
from the program (Kalisch & Kalisch, 2004). In the training schools dur
ing the 1880s and 1890s, physicians gave lectures to probationers on nursing theory, usually in the late evenings after dinner between hospital work
shifts. Superintendents and their assistants taught all of the hands-on nursing practice (Kalisch & Kalisch, 2004).

Probationers (nicknamed "probies") were expected to work 7 days a
week, 70–90 hours a week, during the entire training period. While probationers could often make it through 1 year of this grueling schedule,
3 years of such training took a heavy physical and mental toll that caused
excessive illness and dropout rates (Andrist et al., 2006; Kalisch & Kalisch,
2004). "Isabel Hampton, a pioneer in nursing education, warned that if
schools increased the training period [from 1 year to 3 years], they had to
limit the workday to 8 hours. Her words fell on deaf ears. Physicians, hospital administrators, and the nurse superintendents argued that the 8-hour
workday would be the demise of hospitals" (Andrist et al., 2006, p. 10), and
so the 70–90 hour workweek continued. This issue was not substantively
addressed again until 1928, when a study of nurse training schools entitled
Nurses, Patients, and Pocketbooks, was completed and published by May

Ayers Burgess, a member of the Committee on the Grading of Nursing Schools. A major finding of this study was that the vast majority of nursing schools still required students to work more than 40 hours a week, even though the 40-hour workweek was standard in most other industries and occupations in the United States by this time (Andrist et al., 2006).

Minority nurses found limited educational opportunities. The first Black nursing school graduate in the United States was Mary P. Mahoney, who completed a course of study at New England Hospital for Women and Children in 1879. The first nursing school established solely for Black women was founded at Spelman Seminary in Atlanta, Georgia in 1879. Two other schools devoted to educating Black nurses were established at Hampton Institute in Virginia, and at Providence Hospital in Chicago in 1891 (Hine, 1989; Kalisch & Kalisch, 2004).

Five schools of nursing for men were opened in the United States during the late 1800s (O'Lynn & Tranbarger, 2007):

- In 1886, a school for male nurses opened in Blackwell's Welfare Island, New York.
- In 1886, McLean Hospital School of Nursing for Men opened in Waverley, Massachusetts.
- In 1888, Mills School of Nursing for Men opened in Bellevue Hospital in New York City.
- In 1888, St. Vincent Hospital School for Men opened in New York City.
- In 1898, the Alexian Brothers Hospital School of Nursing opened in Chicago, Illinois.

The nurse training schools that were opened for men and Black women followed the Nightingale training school model, similar to most other nurse training schools in the United States.

Advances in Practice

IN THE EARLY TO MIDDLE 1800s, healthcare practices were similar to those in Colonial times. There was little understanding about how the human body worked, how infection was spread, or what could be done to significantly aid healing for illnesses and injury, or to protect and assist childbearing women. Apothecaries sold medicines that were often harmful to unsuspecting patents. Many quack treatments for illness and injury were available from itinerant salesmen or by mail order, and these proved to be at best ineffective and at worst harmful or lethal (Kalisch & Kalisch, 2004). Fortunately, in the 1880s and 1890s, several advancements in knowledge related to health care provided means for effective assessment and treatment of a variety of ailments and formed the underpinnings of modern healthcare practices.

Ether was successfully used by American doctor J. Collins Warren to anesthetize a surgical patient in 1846. In 1847, James Y. Simpson, a Scottish obstetrician, successfully used chloroform to anesthetize women in childbirth. After the work of these two physicians became known, anesthetizing surgical patients with ether or chloroform rapidly became common practice in Europe and the United States, thereby revolutionizing surgical procedures by allowing surgeons to work more carefully, and to perform more complex procedures that were previously impossible (Kalisch & Kalisch, 2004).

During the early and mid-1800s, physicians prided themselves on the amount of old and new blood encrusted on their clothing, aprons, and hands as they went from one patient visit to the next. Realizing that previously healthy new mothers became ill with childbed fever (obstetrical infection) after being examined by obstetricians who had come directly from performing postmortem exams, Ignaz Philipp Semmelweis, a Viennese obstetrician, conveyed the theory that unseen germs from human body fluids caused infections. He asserted that simple hand washing would decrease postpartum deaths from childbed fever. Amidst great protest from others, he required obstetricians working for him in obstetrical hospital wards to wash their hands in a solution of chlorine before examining each patent. Between 1846 and 1848, this simple action reduced the death rate in his maternity wards by 90%. Even though a documented drop in maternal deaths validated Semmelweis's observations, peers ridiculed his work and refused to believe the findings. He tried to convince the medical community that simple hand washing could save the lives of countless childbearing women, but he could not convince others of this. Eventually, he lost his sanity and died in an asylum (Kalisch & Kalisch, 2004). Twenty years after Semmelweis initially proposed the concept, Joseph Lister successfully

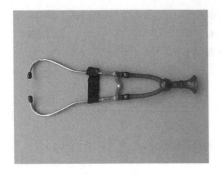

Stethoscope, circa 1800s

convinced the medical community that unseen germs could cause infection. Physicians and surgeons began to accept the germ theory of infection, and began using antiseptics to decrease the likelihood of infection. The practices of antisepsis and asepsis, i.e., cleaning and/or sterilization of hands, clothes, instruments, dressings, etc., became commonplace in the late 1800s. In 1891, William Halsted of Baltimore introduced the use of rubber gloves (Kalisch & Kalisch, 2004).

Many diagnostic instruments were introduced in the 1800s, which significantly improved diagnostic consistency and accuracy. A few of the more notable instruments were (Kalisch & Kalisch, 2004):

- Stethoscopes to listen to the heart, lungs, and bowels
- Thermometers to measure body temperature
- Hypodermic needles to inject medications
- Opthalmoscopes to assess the eyes
- Laryngoscopes to assess the throat and larynx
- Sphygmomanometers to measure blood pressure
- Cystoscopes to assess the bladder
- Bronchoscopes to assess the lungs
- X-ray machines to view the interior of the body

There were also many advancements in bacteriology and immunology in the late 1800s. Scientists and physicians used improved microscopes to identify common infectious agents like *Haemophilus influenzae* and *E. coli*, and those that caused gonorrhea, leprosy, anthrax, typhoid fever, malaria, tuberculosis, diphtheria, tetanus, which led the way for improved diagnosis and treatment. Louis Pasteur developed a vaccine for anthrax in 1881, paving the way for later creation of vaccines for a number of infections, including rabies in 1885. The importance of the discovery of vaccines in the 1800s cannot be underestimated in relation to the management of common human diseases. Present-day vaccine research and development remains vigorous and ongoing.

All of these advances in health care had a profound effect on nursing education and nursing care. Nurses began learning more about how the human body functioned, particularly in relation to infection. Nurses learned to use many new diagnostic instruments. They began participating in surgeries and treatments using antisepsis and asepsis, and they became responsible for setting up and maintaining aseptic operating rooms and treatments. Nurses began administering anesthetic agents to surgical patients and were often the primary providers of anesthetics during surgeries. Overall, patient outcomes improved as nurses and other healthcare providers became more adept at creating and using new technologies. Nurses were faced with continual change, increased responsibility, and rapid technological advancement. Though outward appearances differ significantly, today's nurses must cope with the same basic issues that nurses faced in the late 1800s related to the brisk development and real-world application of new technologies.

War and Its Effects on Nursing

THOUGH LITTLE HISTORICAL INFORMATION IS available about nursing in the War of 1812, the Indian Wars, or the Mexican War, it is safe to assume that nursing care for wounded and ill soldiers was similar to what was found in the Revolutionary War; i.e., few paid and/or trained nurses available and untrained people providing the bulk of the care at the front lines. Nursing activities during the Civil War and the Spanish-American War are discussed here.

The Civil War (1861–1865) was the largest of the five wars fought by Americans during the 1800s and resulted in the death of roughly 618,000 men (Brinkley, 2003; Kalisch & Kalisch, 2004). When the Civil War began, formal training for nurses was only an obscure concept; however, lessons from the Crimean War and Florence Nightingale had made it clear to Americans that nurses (even if they were untrained) were needed in times of war to care for wounded and ill soldiers. Scores of northern women offered their services to provide nursing care to Union soldiers at the beginning of the war. One hundred women were selected to take a special short course in nursing (taught by New York physicians) and then sent to the front lines under the direction of Dorothea Lynde Dix (Kalisch & Kalisch, 2004). Dix, though not

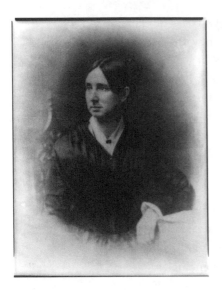

Dorothea Lynde Dix

a nurse, was a well-known humanitarian who worked on behalf of humane treatment for the mentally ill in the United States during the mid- to late 1800s. Dix was given the responsibility of organizing a corps of female nurses to serve Union soldiers throughout the Civil War. She eventually appointed 3,214 army nurses who were sent to various battlefronts and received weekly pay and rations from the United States government for their efforts (Kalisch & Kalisch, 2004).

The work of Florence Nightingale had begun to improve the image of nursing; however, nursing was still viewed by many as inappropriate work for respectable women. Even though nurses were formally recruited, dispatched, and financially compensated by the American government in the Civil War, they were often ridiculed and not supported in their efforts by military officers and physicians. At the same time, infantrymen who received nursing care expressed gratitude and appreciation (Donahue, 1996: Kalisch & Kalisch, 2004). This situation was similar to Nightingale's experiences in the Crimean War.

Despite the commission of Dix to organize nursing efforts in the Civil War, she was unable to exert widespread control and nursing remained, for the most part, in utter disarray. People who acted as nurses were society women, wives of generals, middle-class housewives, destitute paupers, sisters, friends, either paid or unpaid, and sometimes qualified or wholly unqualified (Sarnecky, 1997). "In short, although many urged and some tried to implement standards of selection and periods of training for nurses, the Union nursing corps nonetheless remained a motley group of women who shared little more than their lack of qualifications" (Kalisch & Kalisch, 2004, p. 45).

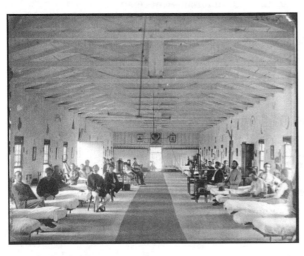

Patients in Ward K of Armory Square Hospital, Washington, D.C., circa 1862–1865

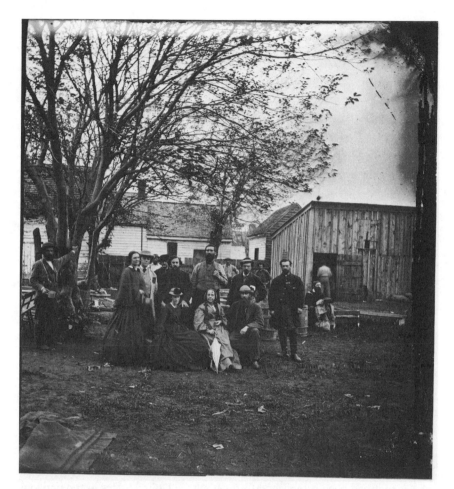

Nurses and Offices of the U.S. Sanitary Commission in Fredericksburg, Virginia, 1864

In the South, though a few hardy and persistent women provided nursing care at the front lines, men opposed the presence of female nurses to such an extent that most of the nursing duties fell upon Confederate infantrymen who were recovering from wounds themselves. Women who dared to enter military hospitals in the South with the intent of providing nursing care were treated with disrespect and animosity by the military officers and physicians, and they were met with dismay by southern civilians who viewed nursing to be entirely inappropriate for respectable women (Sarnecky, 1997).

Military nursing during the Civil War was not a rousing success, in either the North or the South, in terms of advancement for the American nursing

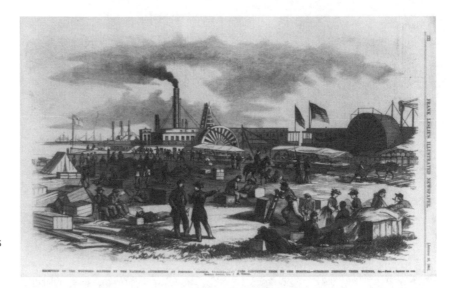

"Reception of the wounded soldiers by the national authorities at Fortress Monroe, Virginia," 1862

profession as a whole. The soldiers who benefited from the care of trained nurses were vocal in their appreciation, and this likely helped to increase public appreciation for the usefulness of trained nurses, much as it had in England after the work of Nightingale and her trained nurses in Crimea. After the war was over, several women who had worked as nurses at the front lines took leading roles in the establishment of nurse training schools in the United States (Kalisch & Kalisch, 2004).

The Spanish-American War (1989–1902) resulted in the creation of an Army Nurse Corps consisting *only* of nurse graduates from nearly 200 nurse training schools that had been established throughout the United States in the previous 40 years. This was the first time in American history that trained nurses were fully accepted into military hospitals (Donahue, 1996; Kalisch & Kalisch, 2004). Nurses were stationed in military hospitals in the United States, Puerto Rico, Cuba, Hawaii, the Philippine Islands, and on a hospital ship named the *USS Relief* (Donahue, 1996).

The United States was poorly prepared for the Spanish-American War, and this was reflected in the dismally disorganized and undersupplied military hospitals on all fronts (Sarnecky, 1997). Upon arrival at their assigned hospitals, nurses were confronted with filth, disarray, and rampant malaria, dysentery, typhoid, and yellow fever. Mismanagement of the troops caused inordinately high numbers of soldiers to die from disease rather than battle wounds. "May 1898 through April 1899, the army suffered 968 battle casualties and 5438 deaths from disease." (Kalisch & Kalisch, 2004, p. 155)

In response to the large numbers of soldiers infected with typhoid and yellow fever, American army physicians conducted research to determine mode of transmission for these two diseases. Nurses and physicians often volunteered to be experimental subjects as researchers worked to identify the causes and vectors. It was determined that flies and unclean practices caused the spread of typhoid fever. A team of physicians in Cuba determined that common house mosquitoes carried yellow fever and that human beings were infected by the bite of infected mosquitoes and *not* by exposure to other infected human beings. A nurse by the name of Clara Maass, who was stationed in Cuba, was the last experimental subject to die of yellow fever after volunteering to be bitten on two separate occasions by mosquitoes known to be carrying the disease. Maass was the only woman and the only American to die during the yellow fever experiments. In 1976, the United States issued a commemorative stamp in honor of her great sacrifice (Donahue, 1996).

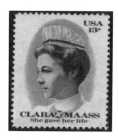

Clara Maass stamp, issued August 18, 1976

The Spanish-American War resulted in advancement for the profession of nursing in the United States because it prompted the first formal large-scale effort to recruit trained nurses for military service in wartime. The army nurse corps that was established during this war paved the way for future military nursing. "The war experience definitely proved the superiority of the trained nurse over the untrained volunteer and led to the initiation of a permanent nurse corps" for the American military (Donahue, 1996, p. 288).

Nursing Workforce Issues

WITH THE OPENING OF NURSE training schools in American hospitals, hospital administrators saw a way to economically staff hospitals with nursing students (Donahue, 1996; Kalisch & Kalisch, 2004). Hospital-based nurse training schools proliferated, and there was no shortage of applicants. Although pay for graduate nurses was inadequate to supply basic human needs, it was often higher for nursing than for other jobs available to women during this time period, which made it an attractive option for women trying to support themselves.

> In 1888, the Department of Labor investigated the weekly wages paid to women in 22 large cities. It found the average weekly wages varied from a high of $6.91 in San Francisco to a low of $3.93 in Richmond.... A government report noted that this was hardly enough to buy the necessities of life. (Kalisch & Kalisch, 2004, p. 136)

On the other hand, graduate nurses working in private duty settings might earn between $10.00 and $40.00 per week, depending on the difficulty of the case. These higher earnings were offset by some harsh realities. Private duty nurses worked 24 hours a day, 7 days a week while on a case; there were often long gaps of time between cases (when a nurse earned no money at all), and it was sometimes difficult to collect payment. Still, private duty nursing was considered one of the best jobs for women in the 1880s and 1890s (Kalisch & Kalisch, 2004).

Workforce issues related to minorities in nursing made little progress in the 1800s. As the Nightingale model of nursing took hold in the United States, nursing became more acceptable for one group (White, conservative, middle-class women) while becoming less acceptable for all of the others. Black women found it difficult to gain admission to nurse training schools because there were racial quotas in the North and segregation laws in the South. There were few nurse training schools devoted to educating Black women as nurses and health care for Black Americans suffered due to lack of qualified nurses and other healthcare providers (Hine, 1989). Opportunities for men in nursing were also limited as the public began to strongly equate nursing with middle-class White women. The limited opportunities for men in nursing that existed in relation to gender-segregated hospital wards disappeared as women became the only accepted caregivers in hospital settings. Nightingale model nurse training schools did not accept men at all and there was a paucity of nurse training schools for men (O'Lynn & Tranbarger, 2007). While opportunity greeted one group, exclusion and discrimination greeted all of the others.

Licensure and Regulation

NURSE TRAINING SCHOOLS CONTINUED TO keep rolls of graduate nurses who could be referred for private duty nursing assignments.

There was still no formal licensure or regulation of nursing practice in the United States.

Nursing Research

NURSES IN THE 1800S RELIED, for the most part, on tradition to guide practice. Nursing education in the newly formed nurse training schools was based on widely accepted practices that had not been validated by research findings. Scientific breakthroughs during the 1800s helped to improve nursing practice indirectly as nurses altered interventions based on new knowledge generated by scientists and physicians. There is no record of an organized effort among nurses to generate research-based knowledge aimed at clarifying whether or not specific nursing practices resulted in measurably effective patient outcomes.

Summary

THE 1800S IN THE UNITED States were turbulent and encompassed sweeping sociopolitical upheaval and change. During this 100-year span, nursing transitioned from an unacceptable pursuit to a preferred occupation for unmarried, White, middle-class women. The United States participated in five wars during this time period, and nurses participated in them all to varying degrees, but never in a fully organized way until the Spanish-American War, when an army nurse corps made up entirely of graduate nurses was formed. The graduate nurses came from newly established American nurse training schools modeled after Nightingale's nurse training schools in Great Britain. These schools did not admit men, and they only admitted a limited number of Black female students. A few training schools for minorities were opened, but the vast majority of graduate nurses in the United States at this time were White, middle-class women, and this remains the norm today. Nursing education and practice changed dramatically between the beginning and end of the century as scientific discoveries related to health care transformed care delivery in relation to anesthetics, antisepsis, asepsis, advancement of diagnostic instruments, and vaccine development. There were no significant developments during this time related to nursing licensure, regulation, and research; however, increased public acceptance and the advent of organized nursing education set the stage for the emergence of nurse leaders who ushered in a new level of professionalism.

⬥ IDEAS FOR FURTHER EXPLORATION

1. Learn more about any of the five wars that the United States engaged in during the 1800s, which included the War of 1812, the Indian Wars, the Mexican War, the Civil War, and the Spanish-American War.

2. Assess the proportion of men and ethnic/racial minorities in nursing in the United States by searching for this information on the United States Bureau of Labor Statistics Web site. How is the United States doing in relation to diversity among nurses? How might we go about attracting and retaining more minorities into the nursing profession?

3. The 19th century is often referred to as the golden age of medicine because of multiple scientific discoveries related to health care that occurred during this era. Research historical records to learn about discoveries not discussed in this text. Consider how these discoveries have impacted nursing practice.

⫸ DISCUSSION QUESTIONS: APPLICATION TO CURRENT PRACTICE

1. Inordinately low pay in relation to the level of education, training, responsibility, and risk that accompanies nursing work has been of concern to many nurses since the 1800s. Do you consider this an issue today? Why or why not?

2. The Nightingale training schools helped to establish professional nursing in the United States; however, they also resulted in the exclusion of men from nursing. Consider a nursing work environment that you have participated in as a patient, a student, or a professional nurse. Identify and describe any remnants of the Nightingale model of nursing that you observed. (There are still many in virtually every nursing environment.) Are men still excluded in any way in nursing work environments? How? By whom? What might you do to minimize and/ or eliminate the exclusion of men that still occurs in various aspects of nursing practice?

3. Though outward appearances differ significantly, today's nurses must cope with the same basic issues that nurses faced in the late 1800s related to the brisk development and real-world application of new technologies. Rapid change seems to be a continuing theme in nursing, starting at the very beginning of the establishment of nursing in America, persisting today, and likely to remain a concern in the future. Do you embrace or resist workplace change? Explain your answer using examples from a past work experience (nonnursing examples are okay to describe). Identify and describe three strategies for coping with change that would be helpful for today's nurses.

✦ MeSH SEARCH TERMS

American Civil War
Schools, nursing
Spanish-American War, 1898

✦ SUGGESTED READING

Alcott, L. M. & Parsons, E. E. (1984). *Civil War nursing*. New York: Garland.

Ashley, J. A. (1976). *Hospitals, paternalism, and the role of the nurse*. New York: Teachers College Press.

Franklin, R. (2005). *The Nightingale sisters: The making of a nurse in 1800's America*. West Sussex, UK: Diggory Press.

Maher, M. D. (1989). *To bind up the wounds: Catholic sister nurses in the U.S. Civil War*. New York: Greenwood Press.

Potgeier, E. (1992). *Professional nursing education, 1860–1991*. Pretoria: Academica.

Thoms, A. B. (1985). *Pathfinders: A history of the progress of colored graduate nurses*. New York: Garland.

✦ REFERENCES

Andrist, L. C., Nicholas, P. K., & Wolf, K. A. (Eds.). (2006). *A history of nursing ideas.* Sudbury, MA: Jones and Bartlett.

Brinkley, A. (2003). *American history: A survey.* (11th ed.). New York: McGraw-Hill.

Collins, G. (2003). *America's women: 400 years of dolls, drudges, helpmates, and heroines.* New York: William Morrow.

D'Antonio, P., Baer, E. D., Rinker, S. D., & Lynaugh, J. E. (Eds.). (2007). *Nurses' work: Issues across time and place.* New York: Springer.

Donahue, M. P. (1996). *Nursing: The finest art* (2nd ed.). St. Louis: Mosby.

Hine, B. C. (1989). *Black women in white: Racial conflict and cooperation in the nursing profession.* Bloomington: Indiana University Press.

Houweling, L. (2004). Image, function, and style: A history of the nursing uniform. *American Journal of Nursing, 104*(4), 40–48.

Kalisch, P. A. & Kalisch, B. J. (2004). *American nursing: A history* (4th ed.). Philadelphia: Lippincott, Williams, and Wilkins.

O'Lynn, C. E., & Tranbarger, R. E. (Eds.). (2007). *Men in nursing: History, challenges, and opportunities.* New York: Springer

Sarnecky, M. T. (1997). Nursing in the American army from the Revolution to the Spanish-American War. *Nursing History Review, 5,* 49–69.

United States Department of Veteran's Affairs (2007). *America's wars fact sheet.* Washington, DC: Office of Public Affairs.

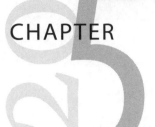

Nursing in the United States From 1900 to the Early 1920s

1901
- Clara Maass dies after participating in research on yellow fever
- Theodore Roosevelt elected president
- Army Nurse Corps founded

1905
American Journal of Nursing published for the first time

1907
Navy Nurse Corps developed

1909
- First nursing school program associated with a university founded
- National Association for the Advancement of Colored People (NAACP) founded

| 1900 | 1901 | 1902 | 1903 | 1904 | 1905 | 1906 | 1907 | 1908 | 1909 |

1900
- Walter Reed proves yellow fever is caused by mosquito bites
- Mary Adelaide Nutting introduces science and theory prior to clinical practice

1902
Lillian Wald forms New York public school nursing program

1906
San Francisco earthquake rescue efforts involve national public health services

1908
National Association of Colored Graduate Nurses is formed

A NEW CENTURY BRINGS NOVEL IDEAS AND SOCIAL CONCERNS

Deborah M. Judd

1911
Nurse's Associated Alumnae of the United States and Canada becomes the American Nurses Association (ANA)

1913
- Panama Canal opens
- R. J. Reynolds sells the first cigarettes

1917–1918   Spanish flu epidemic kills over 20 million

| 1910 | 1911 | 1912 | 1913 | 1914 | 1915 | 1916 | 1917 | 1918 | 1919 | 1920 |

1910
Florence Nightingale dies

1912
- The Society of Superintendents of Training Schools becomes the National League for Nursing Education (NLN)
- Children's Bureau established; promotes welfare of children, addresses child labor issues
- National Organization for Public Health Nursing is formed

1914
Margaret Sanger opens a clinic for birth control

1914–1918   World War I

1920
19th Amendment ratified, allows women to vote

1910–1912   Isabel Hampton Robb promotes educational reform

OUR NURSING HERITAGE: KEY PEOPLE

Annie Damer	Member of the early nursing organizations
	Private duty nurse involved in the tuberculosis public health program
	Early nurse examiner for licensure, promoted nurse credentialing
Mary E.P. Davis	Managed the *American Journal of Nursing*
	Promoted nursing as more than "cheap labor"
Jane Delano	Served as president of the Nurses' Associated Alumnae
	Served as superintendent of the Army Nurse Corps
	Recruited nurses for the Red Cross Nurse Reserves, helping supply over 20,000 nurses to serve in World War I
Lavinia Lloyd Dock	Bellevue Training School supervisor
	Wrote one of the first nursing textbooks—*Materia Medica for Nurses*
	Served as secretary of the International Council of Nurses (ICN)
Martha Minerva Franklin	Only Black graduate of her class at the Woman's Hospital Training School
	Organized the National Association for Colored Graduate Nurses
	Promoted racial equality in nursing
Annie Goodrich	Served as New York State Inspector for Training Schools
	1st dean of Yale Graduate School of Nursing
	Served as dean of the Army School of Nursing
Stella Goostray	Served as secretary for the National League for Nursing Education
	Served on the *American Journal of Nursing* board
	Committee on the Grading of Nursing Schools nurse consultant
Lucille Elizabeth Notter	Nurse researcher who worked to develop the journal *Nursing Research*
	Authored *Professional Nursing: Foundations, Perspectives, and Relationships*
	Was a visiting nurse for over 10 years

Clara Noyes	Director of the American Red Cross Bureau of Nursing, prepared nurses for World War I
	Promoted child welfare work
	Post-war recommendations had an international impact on hospitals, public health, and education
Mary Adelaide Nutting	Advocate for educational reform and university education for nurses
	Author of several nursing texts and guides
	First professor of nursing
Mary D. Osborne	Promoted maternal and child health and prenatal care
	Regulated "granny" midwives, instituted midwife training
Sophia Palmer	First editor of the *American Journal of Nursing*
	Promoted state registration of nurses
	Charter member of the American Nurses Association and The American Society of Superintendents of Training Schools for Nurses
Mabel Keaton Staupers	Promoted racial equality in both nursing and healthcare provision
	Wrote *No Time for Prejudice*
	Served on the Harlem Tuberculosis Committee
Julia Catherine Stimson	First female major in the Army; superintendent of the Army Nurse Corps; dean of the Army School of Nursing
	Chief nurse of the American Red Cross during World War I
	Served as president of the American Nurses Association
Adah Belle Thoms	Encouraged equality for Black nurses and student nurses
	Served as superintendent of the Lincoln School for Nurses
	Promoted Black nurse participation in the Red Cross

Sociopolitical Climate

BY THE CLOSE OF THE 19th century, millions of immigrants had entered the United States through Ellis Island. From the 1880s until 1910, the demographic of immigrant populations changed such that there were more individuals from eastern Europe and the Mediterranean gathering along the eastern shores of the United States than there were from England, Scandinavia, or western Europe (Kalisch & Kalisch, 2004). On the Pacific Coast, the harbor of San Francisco welcomed immigrants from the Orient, primarily from Japan and China, although some European immigrants traveled around the cape to find their fortunes. Those wishing for a better life and many opportunities for success came to the United States with limited resources, inadequate preparation, and unrealistic expectations for what they would find once they arrived in the land of promise. These great shifts in population resulted in major health issues, economic dilemmas, and a general lack of support for the newly arrived citizens.

"Cities, ill prepared to cope with rapid growth, were governed inadequately and often dishonestly by politicians whose base of support lay in wards populated by immigrants inexperienced with American politics and grateful for services provided by the 'machine'" (Kerber & De Hart, 1995, p. 228). Populations in major cities on the East Coast grew at phenomenal rates; housing shortages, sanitation issues, increased disease morbidity, significant mortality, new social problems, and labor concerns related to children and women caused distress for many. Tenement housing became the standard in the cities, and with continued immigration into the United States, issues arose related to changes in ethnicity, substantial poverty, mediocre management of frontier borders, and inability to deal with the significant influx of individuals into a system not adequately prepared to receive them. Worry about the welfare of women and children created an environment for social, economic, and political reform. The Industrial Revolution continued to promote economic growth for the nation while ultimately undermining certain aspects of society. The government was not prepared to adequately deal with rapid immigration, modernization, and the problems or changes in society associated with progressivism. Some felt that because there were no responses to the social issues, that leaders were inefficient and perhaps submissive to those who could wield power because of their status in business or society. Even though the need for social reform was obvious, some professed that elected officials and others who could initiate change did not deal with the most important issues (Brinkley, 2003).

Distinctions in class became more obvious. A limited number of individuals and families who achieved great profit and benefit created monopolies and economic empires, while concerns for the lower- and middle-class members of society expanded. The Department of Commerce and Labor was created in 1903, and many antitrust issues were addressed as the government intervened in national economics. In 1907 a recession arose, and public financial concerns escalated until 1914, when the Federal Trade Commission was formed to resolve further antitrust issues. Political and social reforms were initiated by the rise of Theodore Roosevelt to the presidency of the United States in 1901 after the assassination of President William McKinley (Brinkley, 2003).

Events during this 20-year period of time influenced society and nursing reformation in particular over the next several decades. The National Association for the Advancement of Colored People was founded in 1909. The Constitution was modified such that senators were elected by popular vote when the Seventeenth Amendment was ratified in 1913. The following year, the Panama Canal opened, providing opportunities for better worldwide trade options. Meanwhile, across the Atlantic, there was unrest in many countries. The Bolshevik Revolution occurred in Russia when Germany invaded France and Austria occupied Serbia. World War I began in 1914, and the Treaty of Versailles was not signed until 1919. There were many who were concerned about neutrality and involvement in war as the United States emerged as a world power and assumed greater responsibilities related to foreign policy and influence (Brinkley, 2003; Kalisch & Kalisch, 2004; Mosby, Inc., 2000). Reforms continued through the successive presidencies of William Taft and Woodrow Wilson. Eleanor Roosevelt, the first lady, was actively engaged in social improvements and encouraged many aspects of feminism. Prohibition was established when the Eighteenth Amendment was adopted in 1919, in part due to concerns of many citizens who felt that liquor had a negative influence on society and the family. Women's suffrage escalated and was no longer just a state concern. With the passage of the Nineteenth Amendment in 1920, women were granted certain rights, including the right to vote and the right to own property.

Finally, as women adopted roles that were not the traditional roles of wife and mother, many were concerned about the ultimate effect it would have on the individual, the community, and the nation. This reaction prompted many women and some men to crusade for change in a world that needed progressive thoughts and actions in order to solve social concerns pertaining to health, education, sanitation, violence, sexual responsibility, morals, and economics (Kerber & De Hart, 1995, p. 229). A number of societies and associations emerged, permitting women to influence policy in their communities and eventually the nation. According to Kerber and De Hart, these new organizations allowed women to gain access to politicians,

Nursing Services Club

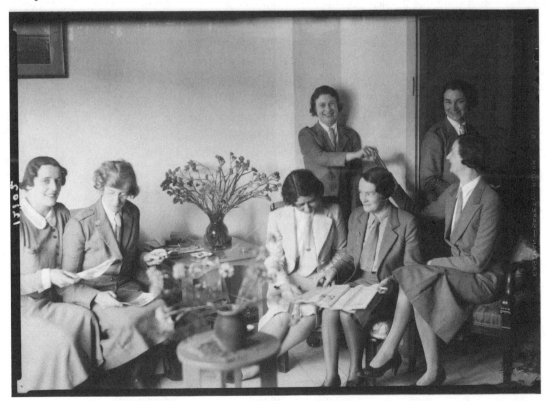

influence society through marches and rallies, and finally influence men, who, at the time, controlled society (p. 229). Some of these organizations included the Women's Christian Temperance Union, the Young Women's Christian Association, the Settlement House Movement, the National Child Labor Committee, the General Federation of Women's Clubs, and the Pure Food Association. Each of these groups and similar social clubs eventually influenced society as they allowed issues of the day to be openly addressed. During the next several decades, social reforms and concerns expressed during this era contributed to many advances for women and children. Female leaders of the day had great foresight and determination to initiate changes that would positively affect women's vocations over the next 50 years.

The Image of Nursing

AS NURSE RESPECTABILITY INCREASED, MANY still believed that the nurses of the day should only be associated with the emerging hospital systems and their judicious control. Nurses' lives were influenced in essence by the hospital schools that accepted, trained, and eventually employed them; their duties and responsibilities were the direct result of the needs in these individual organizations at the turn of the century. Nursing supervisors and physicians of the day determined their attire, the scope of their activities, and their schedules. Nurses just prior to the war had a distinct appearance. In 1916 a standard public uniform was proposed for American Nurses Association (ANA) members appearing in public activities "in which nurses have been given a conspicuous place, as those for preparedness or equal suffrage" ("The Need of a Standard Uniform," 1916, p. 966). Nurses enjoyed a positive image during this time since they represented all things that were good and socially acceptable. Since the uniform represented who they were and their service to society, it was only to be worn while on duty and caring for the public in whatever setting they worked (Houweling, 2004). Because of this belief, which continued into the end of the 20th century, nurses were expected to continue to protect their image by wearing the uniform of their day only while working.

Nursing service was still considered by most to be a Christian characteristic, and thus images of the Victorian era remained associated with the nursing vocation until about 1910 (Houweling, 2004). The attire of a nurse included a basic, clean, modest dress without obvious areas of wear and the traditional apron. Most wore a cap or hat that was unique to the hospital where the nurse had trained as a probie. Nurses were required to present themselves on time, with all details of their appearance determined by the hospital or school in order, and then were evaluated by patients, supervisors, and the attending physicians. Hospital nurses continued to train and work in their respective facilities, serving patients who often were admitted for extended periods of time.

Mosby, Inc. (2000) summarizes Minnie Goodnow's (1919) description of nurses:

> Work was considered an opportunity, since the ordinary female could nurse and those that could be trained were deemed able to acquire the techniques and characteristics necessary for "the spirit of her art" ... All were to bear in mind that you should be ready and willing to do your best and even more than required without emotions that would betray your feelings ... One was not to appear hurried or without interest in the patient or the doctor, while maintaining appropriate but socially acceptable relationships with all; be considerate, do not contradict, please others, be honest, consider the patient's wellbeing, don't judge based on social status, and never forget that it is your "good breeding and teachableness" that allow you to serve others as a probationer and eventually a nurse. (p. 11)

The development of complex communities that were crowded and impoverished allowed nurses to offer expanded nursing services to those who needed them but were not eligible for hospital stays or physician care. As home and clinic health services expanded, the image of a visiting or home nurse was likely to include a modest and simple dress with a fitted bodice, long sleeves and a white smock; the collar was high, and all nurses wore a black or white hat. Eventually they adopted a blue uniform, which allowed others to recognize them as a public health nurse. Because these nurses did not work in the hospital setting, they carried a black bag that held their supplies to be used when administering to the sick or injured.

It was not uncommon for nurses who rendered care in such circumstances to go directly into the community and live and work with their patients and families. Their uniform not only identified who they were but also offered them some protection in areas where they might otherwise feel unsafe. Services provided by these early school or home health nurses included checking on the status of children in or out of school, delivering babies, providing education and protection to those less fortunate, educating individuals unfamiliar with certain aspects of personal hygiene or disease, and monitoring patient progress. Most times the nurse not only cared for a specific patient but also the extended family unit.

Almost all nurses were female during this era; there were only four male nursing schools and very few others admitted males into the realms of their nurse training programs. Since nurses were female, the style of the uniform was in keeping with conservative societal trends for a single female. Depending on the location of service, a nurse might vary her uniform to fit the circumstances, such as horseback riding for the frontier or town and country nursing services. Nurses might also alter their uniforms to fit the climate and the socioeconomic status of the patients they cared for in order to fit into the community they serviced. Since nurses basically lived and worked in the same setting, their entire existence was an image that society knew and understood.

The Education of Nurses

IN THE EARLY 1900s, EDUCATION for nurses continued to change as a result of recommendations from the American Society of Superintendents of Training Schools for Nurses. Various committees worked together to ensure that nurses were prepared for leadership under the auspices of Isabel Hampton Robb. Teachers College and Columbia University became model schools for nursing education.

> Nursing education should find its place in the university, which is another way of saying that it belongs where all educational expressions have been increasingly placed, and for the reason that universal knowledge is there ... [for] the needs of the students as future builders of the community. (Goodrich, 1932, p. 173)

As nurse leaders better understood the need for academic knowledge as well as clinical knowledge, a group of nurses at Teacher's College began to include an emphasis on nursing experiences, phases of nurse education,

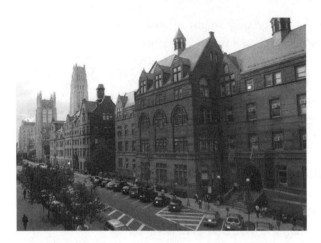

Teacher's College,
Columbia University

clinical training, socialization into the hospital program, supervision, teaching, and a focus on nurse specialties including public health and school nursing in their revised lectures. These leaders knew that hospital school programs of the past would never be able to promote scientific nursing knowledge without the assistance of an academic institution and faculty who were prepared with a scientific background. Prior to that point in time, educators were from the hospital organization or the medical community and taught from a personal perspective with emphasis on the notion that a nurse was to aid the doctor and care for all of the patients' needs while maintaining a sanitary environment suitable for adequate nourishment and healing (Donahue, 1996, pp. 288–289).

As more theory and alternative courses were introduced into the training experiences of nurses, physicians believed that nurses were being taught foolish knowledge, and that too much theory would lead to too little care (Kalisch & Kalisch, 2004). Debate ensued as physicians believed that understanding of unnecessary things would impede the nurses' ability to effectively care for their patients. Nurse leaders, however, felt that additional knowledge would enhance the care the nurses would provide. Educational modification based on theory and the acquisition of scientific knowledge ushered in an era of academic nursing education associated with either a college or a university education.

Within 10 years, Mary Adelaide Nutting, working at Johns Hopkins Hospital, became the first nursing professor and eventually the first nursing chairperson. Nurses of the day, such as Lillian Wald, Mary Brewster, Lina Rogers, Mary Sewell Gardner, Lavinia Lloyd Dock, and others encouraged the addition of specific skills and knowledge to augment the nurturing and housekeeping duties that were traditionally part of most hospital-based nursing practices. They wanted to demonstrate to society the nurse's intellectual capacity and ability to accomplish great things as they "banded together to support educational standards, to set up legal controls to prevent the spread of poor schools, and to prevent unlimited expansion" (Stewart, 1943, p. 129). These nurse leaders, through collaborative efforts, promoted educational reforms that resulted in college- or university-affiliated programs for nurses. The suggested curriculum changes they encouraged continued to be implemented in ways that would impact educational opportunities for all nurses during the entire century as theory inclusion became an integral part of a nurse's training.

Since nursing services were becoming more diversified, there arose a need to educate nurses for a variety of settings. There were many suggestions to improve educational standards and ensure practice regulation. Some of these recommendations included preparation classes, practical courses, science lessons (such as those in anatomy), and specific theory relating to all aspects of patient care, from hygiene to the operating theater. Additionally, probationers were referred to as student nurses, and training superintendents were called nursing teachers or faculty. Mary Roberts Rinehart (1931) describes the obstacles that nurses encountered during their struggle to achieve professionalism in her reflection, *My Story*:

> The simple, plain hell faced by the young nurse is a world so strange and at times so terrible, that even now it hurts to remember it ... By the time I graduated there was no phase of human life or human suffering which I had not touched ... I had no knowledge whatever of brutality, or cruelty, or starvation ... there was born in me something which has never died, a terrible and often devastating pity and compassion, for the weak, the sick and the humble ... these things happen and the world is powerless to prevent them ... I stood one night beside a man who had been [injured]. I wanted him to die quickly ... I can't stand it. Die and stop suffering ... I can't stand it. I can't! When I felt I had suffered, I set up a defensive mechanism; don't think, don't feel. It was automatic. (pp. 45–46 and 65–69)

Nurses today may still feel the same, but through unfathomable technology and discovery, they can and do now change things that were once unchangeable. They have acquired significant amounts of theory about how to care for their patients in the most challenging of conditions, and use their own cognition and power to heal them in ways that only a nurse can.

Advances in Practice

WOMEN WHO WERE GAINING MORE autonomy came together and began to request political recognition and social reforms to alleviate suffering and disparity. Several manuscripts were written describing social conditions, economic injustice, racial concerns, and gender inconsistency. These works and the political progressivism of the time allowed for advancement of the nursing profession. A few notable women became active in political and healthcare reform, and changed conditions for those for whom they advocated when they formed the New York Public School Nursing program in 1902 and the Women's Trade Union in 1903. Through the efforts of Lillian Wald, Mary Brewster, and some of their peers, the Henry Street Settlement and Metropolitan Life Insurance Company established a collaborative relationship for visiting nurse services in Manhattan. Over the next few years, services were expanded into other major metropolitan areas in the Northeast where visiting nurses were active. In each of these areas a Visiting Nurses' Association was formed to establish services with companies for their employees (Kalisch & Kalisch, 2004; Mosby, Inc., 2000).

In 1899, Nutting, along with other notable women (including the wives of several legislators) petitioned for the establishment of a new Army Nurse Corps. It was believed that there would be significant advantage to working for the military since standards of care would be designed specifically for medical and nursing situations associated with war. This proposal was adopted in 1901, during the reorganization of the army, and it eventually led to the development of another military nurse corps known as the Navy Nurse Corps in 1907 (Kalisch & Kalisch, 2004). With the acceptance of these military nurse corps, females replaced male corpsmen as a more efficient use of resources and thus promoted nursing as a female vocation.

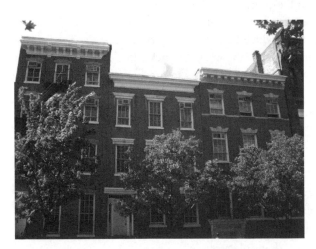

Henry Street Settlement, Manhattan, New York

When nurses entered the community, they did extremely well treating the conditions of the day and connecting with individuals of all socioeconomic and cultural backgrounds. Community successes along with nurses' newfound independence caused concern among some who had had been the main providers of care—district and hospital physicians. Nurses who remained in the hospital under constant supervision of nurse superintendents began to wonder about their role, duties, and abilities to function more independently as their community peers were doing. One physician in the Northeast commented, "the nurse took the temperature, pulse, and respiration, opened the windows and put the pneumonia patient on a milk diet, and left nothing for the physician to do." Another surgeon reported, "they should be prepared for any emergency ... even to giving an intravenous or to re-ligating slipped abdominal sutures" (Foley, 1913, p. 451).

The discussion and debate concerning independent functioning of the individual nurse continued, and in 1912 the scope of visiting nurses was defined when the Chicago Visiting Nurses Association adopted recommendations for care, which became known as standing orders. These orders included descriptions on bathing, diets and nutrition, enemas, environmental conditions, skin and wound treatments, vital signs, relaxation strategies such as rubs, and equipment use, limiting their duties to care without medicine administration, including commonly used items such as castor oil (Kalisch & Kalisch, 2004, p. 169).

In 1895, Lillian Wald ensured life, liberty, and the pursuit of happiness for many as she endeavored to bring the promises of America to those who hoped for a better tomorrow.

> Over broken asphalt, over dirty mattresses and heaps of refuse we went ... There were two rooms and a family of seven not only lived here but shared their quarters with boarders ... [I felt] ashamed of being a part of society that permitted such conditions to exist ...What I had seen had shown me where my path lay. (Jewish Women's Archive, 2008a)

Wald defined nursing care in new ways and made a bold statement along with her colleague, Mary Brewster. They promoted community nursing and tried to ensure that women and children, the poor and the needy, religious immigrants, and new ethnic settlers had an opportunity to receive care when they were sick. More importantly, they insisted that support and education were necessary to prevent disease that often accompanied poverty and crowding.

During the first decade of the 1900s, the school nursing program was introduced, and school nurses became active in caring for children of the community in the schools they attended. Prior to initiation of this program, thousands of students were sent home regularly for any illness, even if it was minor. According to Wald and Lina Rogers, many children were kept from school when they did not need to be, and in other instances disease and contagion were not addressed and communities suffered epidemics (Kalisch & Kalisch, 2004). The school nurses became successful in caring for many diseases of childhood and, more importantly, infections and infestations of the skin such as scabies, ringworm, lice, and skin dermatitis, which were common in the tenements. They accomplished great things as they dealt with social problems and changed the outcomes of many communicable diseases including diarrheal infections, tuberculosis, trachoma, and typhoid fever. They became advocates for the children and their mothers and would often be the only ones who could do so. Florence Kelly (1913) recalls:

> A nurse followed him to his lair and found four brothers and little girl five years old working with incredible rapidity turning out little paper bags ... as come from the grocer.... Not one of the children was tall enough to reach the window sill.... They lived there 18 months in a rear cellar bedroom ... Nobody had visited them but a series of doctors when the children had the diseases of childhood, not one of them had reported them to the truant officer. When the matter was reported to the factory inspector, he said he never knew of anyone occupying that room ... here was a perfectly dead waste, due to the negligence of the physicians who had left everything as it was before.... The two persons who have access everywhere are the nurse and the doctor. (American Academy of Medicine, 1913, pp. 6–7)

Despite the school nurses' achievements in controlling disease and the nuisances of mild illness, in 1906, "excited mothers stormed schools to demand their children [after hearing the rumor] that the children's throats were being cut" (Kalisch & Kalisch, 2004, pp. 167–168). The cause of the riot was in fact due to adenoid operations that had been performed on school premises. Once the mothers were informed of the circumstances their apprehension was alleviated, and over time school nurses became the friends of the community and were trusted to provide necessary services for all (Kalisch & Kalisch, 2004). Even into the mid-1900s, tonsillectomies and adenoidectomies were performed in school settings as a way to control frequent outbreaks of tonsillitis prior to regular use of penicillin antibiotics.

In 1912, Wald prompted Congress to create the United States Children's Bureau after she aroused national attention over the years related to children's health and well-being. She made statements such as the following on many occasions:

> ... the Federal Government concerned itself with the conservation of material wealth, mines and forests, hogs and lobsters, and had long since established bureaus to supply information concerning them, citizens who desired instruction and guidance for the conservation and protection of the children of the nation had no responsible governmental body to which to appeal. (Jewish Women's Archives, 2008b)

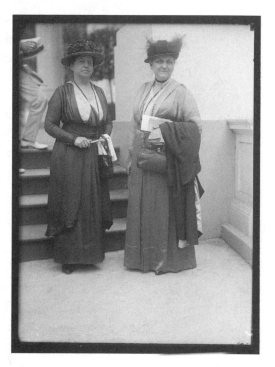

Jane Adams (left) and
Lillian Wald (right)

Under the direction of Julia Lathrop and Grace Abbott, chiefs of the bureau, recommendations and programs were developed related to child labor laws, illegitimate births, juvenile courts, individual state codes for minors, adoption rules and regulations, guardianships, child placements, and offenses against women and children (including sexual abuse). This program has continued to the present and is now part of the Division for Children and Family Services. The bureau not only addressed social issues, but promoted clinics for women and children where services such as prenatal care, postnatal care, and well-child visits/screenings became available (Kalisch & Kalisch, 2004). These programs promoted nurses as the caregiver, and over time their interventions and care decreased morbidity and mortality to these somewhat defenseless populations.

Another nurse reformer, Margaret Sanger, worked to transform women's health as she advocated for education of women regarding pregnancy, sexual activity, birth control, and safer abortion practices. Sanger felt that

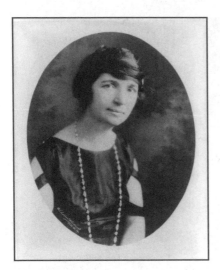

Margaret Sanger

poverty and lack of understanding contributed to health concerns of women in tenements or rural communities or those of society. Many women had multiple births and either lost children or their own lives as a result of the many pregnancies or the practice of self-induced abortion. Sanger wrote a book about her convictions, entitled *The Pivot of Civilization*, which was originally published in 1922.

> We have been criticized for our choice of the term "Birth Control" to express the idea of modern scientific contraception ... the verb "control" means to exercise a directing, guiding, or restraining influence ... Control is guidance, direction, foresight. It implies ... the application of intelligent guidance ... Our effort has been to raise our program from the plane of the emotional to the plane of the scientific ... We must temper our emotion and enthusiasm with the determination of science. (Sanger, 1922, pp. 55–56 and 65)

Sanger worked as a public health nurse in New York City, providing care in maternity cases in a tenement area of the community. She recalls caring for a woman who had attempted an abortion at home to end her pregnancy; this woman recovered after 3 weeks, but a short time later the woman died when she attempted a second abortion and bled to death. As a result of the following experience, Sanger spent the remainder of her life learning about contraception and advocating for medical care and social reforms for women and children.

> When the physician made his last call, he admonished; "Any more such capers, young woman, and there'll be no need to send for me." The convalescent replied, "but what can I do to prevent it?" The physician laughed good-naturedly, "You want to have your cake and eat it too, do you? Well it can't be done. Tell Jake to sleep on the roof." [The woman pleaded with Sanger]: "Tell me the secret and I will never breathe it to a soul." Three months later, the husband called and begged for me to come at once. When I arrived, the wife was in a coma and death followed within minutes. I walked the streets for hours, in years to come I would cite this experience as a turning point in my life. (Sanger, 1922, p. 92)

Technology and Practice

As nurses were perfecting many aspects of care in the hospital and in the community, others were exploring novel ideas and discovering scientific or technological innovations that would soon influence medical and nursing care in this and subsequent eras. From 1900 to 1920, there were several advances that affected care provided to patients well into the 20th century. For example, the source of yellow fever was discovered and verified by Major Walter Reed through the efforts of a nurse who worked with him. Clara Maass actually volunteered to be bitten by a mosquito and eventually gave her life to further knowledge about this disease, which caused more casualties during the Spanish-American War than did the actual combat. Walter Reed Army Hospital near Washington, District of Columbia, was named for him. Also, in 1915, a tuberculosis campaign was promoted by Metropolitan Life Insurance Company to study and eventually prevent its spread, utilizing the health demonstrations, many people were able to participate in this program.

From 1900 to 1920, the following medical advances and discoveries occurred:

- Bayliss and Starling introduced the term *hormone* following their discovery of secretin.
- The first electrocardiogram recording was performed.
- Novocaine (procaine) was used for dental care, and it was eventually tried during medical procedures.
- A test for syphilis was introduced by von Wasserman.
- Blood types were identified by Landsteiner.
- Sir Frederick Hopkins discovered tryptophan and other amino acids, linking nutrition to health.
- Organoscopy (eventually laparoscopy) was developed at Johns Hopkins University Hospital.
- Collodion tubing was used to cleanse the blood, working like an artificial kidney to eliminate toxins (early dialysis). (Mosby, Inc., 2000, pp. 1 and 9)

The first year of the new century ended with an eruption of the bubonic plague in San Francisco, testing the capability of the newly formed United States Public Health Service. Since the organization and headquarters were in the East, there were issues associated with distance and communication. Initially, the presence of the infectious disease was denied and even ignored while rats in the city spread the infection readily in light of poor sanitation and crowding. The disease's spread was believed to be associated with the Chinese immigrant population of the city who were living in deplorable conditions. At one point it seemed that the infection was abating, but with the earthquake and fire of 1906, the disease spread more rapidly, resulting in an epidemic in the Western regions of the country. The Public Health Service became involved and scientists were able to identify the source of the infection and develop strategies to contain it. New knowledge related to vectors and inoculation became available. Programs were initiated to contain the infection, to prevent cargo transportation of rats, and finally to manage the flea population that transmitted the disease from rat to rat, and sometimes from rat to human (United States Public Health Service, 1939).

An epidemic of the Spanish flu killed over 20 million individuals in Europe and Asia by the end of 1917. Even though it was termed the Spanish flu, it was really a very virulent strain of influenza A, which was first noted in Spain during World War I. Some sources say that the flu originated in Tibet, spread into Europe, and by the following year crossed the ocean and emerged on U.S. soil, where it killed over half a million Americans in 1918. This plague killed twice as many people worldwide than did the combat of World War I. The infection affected close to 30% of the population, and affected those who were aged 20–40 years more readily than the young or the elderly. More people died during the winter of 1917–1918 than during the bubonic plague of the 14th century (Billings, 2005).

The American Medical Association (December 28, 1918) released the following statement about the epidemic in the *Journal of the American Medical Association*:

> 1918 has gone: a year momentous as the termination of the most cruel war in the annals of the human race; a year which marked, the end at least for a time, of man's destruction of man; unfortunately a year in which developed a most fatal infectious disease causing the death of hundreds of thousands of human beings. Medical science for four and one-half years devoted itself

to putting men on the firing line and keeping them there. Now it must turn with its whole might to combating the greatest enemy of all—infectious disease ... (Billings, 2005)

"An infection is an act of violence; it is an invasion, a rape, and the body reacts violently" (Barry, 2005, p. 107). According to the physiologist John Hunter, the body's defense lies in its ability to resist putrefaction or infection (Barry, 2005). Hippocrates and Aristotle observed the nature of disease and infection and tried to explain it without actual exploration in about 500 B.C.; Galen wrote his thoughts on medical philosophy around 150 A.D. without invasive investigations. It was a millennium and a half later that Harvey and his peers discovered many new medical ideas. These ideas ushered in an era of new scientific knowledge resulting in novel developments in medicine. Louis Pasteur, Joseph Lister, Robert Koch, and others ascertained much new information about infection, bacteriology, and antisepsis. Their work ultimately affected how nurses and doctors intervened during the influenza epidemic that eventually became a pandemic.

In 1918 Dr. Loring Miner treated a patient who "presented with what seemed common symptoms, although with unusual intensity—violent headache and body aches, high fever, nonproductive cough" (Barry, 2005, p. 93). In a relatively short period of time he saw many others with similar symptoms and diagnosed them with an influenza of severe type, "violent, rapid in its progress through the body, and [often] lethal. [He] contacted the U.S. Public Health Service, but they could not offer assistance nor advice" (Barry, p. 93). Over the next year, many would be affected and eventually strategies for treatment would emerge.

Meanwhile, Paul Lewis, serving in the navy as a physician, had never cared for patients directly since he was a medical scientist.

Within 4 days of his arrival in Philadelphia, 19 sailors were treated for the same infectious disease ... 2 days later 600 were hospitalized with this strange disease; hundreds more sick sailors were sent to a civilian hospital. Lewis took charge and spent hours in his laboratory with all kinds of cultures and specimens, looking for the cause. The infection was so aggressive that doctors and communities could not deal with the sick, the dying, or the dead, and in many communities, people were buried in mass graves in an attempt to control the contagious disease. (Barry, pp. 200–201)

Many other scientists aided in the search for understanding of the infection, and as a result the Rockefeller Institute for Medical Research was founded. From its inception, researchers have added much to the body of knowledge related to infectious diseases. Much of what is now understood about disease processes, pathophysiology, biochemistry, and medical interventions came from their work (Barry, 2005). Through an extensive research process, scientists and doctors were able to develop an immunization to protect people from the flu. Today we still benefit from this knowledge, and annually a vaccine is developed in anticipation of the characteristics of the viral strain that causes it. Eventually medical researchers also developed immunizations and vaccines for other contagious diseases, which, in many cases, led to eradication of the disease in the following decades. At the beginning of the 21st century, many in the United States became negligent in adhering to immunization recommendations, and some diseases, such as pertussis, became problematic again.

In the late 1890s, many new ideas inspired medically-inclined individuals to perfect procedures and equipment, allowing for better patient care during this era. These advancements included the use of sterilizers for surgical equipment, new anesthetics, novel instruments to administer anesthesia, thermometers, X-ray machines, emergency care equipment, gynecological equipment, better blood transfusion techniques, blood pressure monitoring devices, and improved stethoscopes. The desire to enhance patient care with an emphasis on sepsis led to many new procedures and techniques related to surgery primarily, but there were many concepts that emerged, which ultimately affected care of patients who had episodic acute care needs or chronic illnesses. With more focus on patient procedures and ways to cure, nurses and hospitals became more readily available to the average citizen.

War and Its Effects on Nursing

ABOUT 23,000 GRADUATE NURSES WERE appointed to serve during World War I in both the Army and Navy Nurse Corps, with nearly 10,000 of them assigned to overseas duty. Some of these nurses were graduates of the newly established nursing military corps schools. Civilian-trained nurses, along with military-prepared nurses, provided wonderful care despite many challenges. Of those 10,000 military nurses, several received distinguished honors for their courage, valor, and noncombat service; three of them received the second highest military honor, the Distinguished Service award. All of the nurses who received recognition were female despite the fact that there were a few male nurses involved in the conflict. It is reported that only 260 nurses lost their lives during this war, which is less than 1% of the total number of nurses involved in this military effort. The majority of these nurses' deaths were the result of the influenza epidemic in Europe (Mosby, Inc., 2000).

American Red Cross nurses also participated in the care of servicemen in the European theater. Females from society circles paid to be trained by the Red Cross so that they could go overseas to work as nursing aides. Clara Noyes (1917) wrote the following to Nutting:

> There are moments when I wonder whether we can stem the tide and the hysterical desire on the part of thousands, literally thousands, to get into nursing or their hands upon it ... I talk until I am hoarse, dictating letters to doctors and women who want to be Red Cross nurses in a few minutes, not knowing the meaning of the word nurse and what a Red Cross nurse is. (Kalisch & Kalisch, 2004, p. 199)

These American Red Cross nurses eventually became the unauthorized Army Nurse Reserve Corps during World War I.

With an increased need for nurses to serve as military healthcare providers, many were concerned about overall nursing resources and the nation's ability to maintain adequately prepared nurses for both military and civilian hospitals. The Committee on Nursing was established under the direction of the General Medical Board of the U.S. Council for National Defense in order to address nursing supply, general aspects of providing

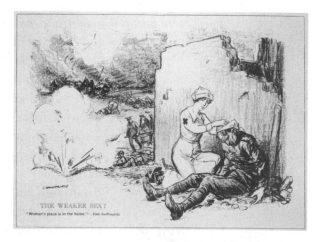

"The Weaker Sex? 'Woman's place is in the home.' —Anti-Suffragists." Red Cross nurse bandages a wounded soldier on the battlefield

health care, specific education related to military nursing, and to finally improve the care of soldiers related to lessons learned from the Civil War and the Spanish-American War. Requirements for applicants, personal qualifications, and educational recommendations were determined by this committee. As was still the norm for noncivilian nurses, military nurses had to be single, ages 25 to 35, and trained in a facility that had at least 100 beds (Kalisch & Kalisch, 2004).

Nurses serving in hospitals on U.S. soil cared for wounded or ill soldiers who had been stabilized by military nurses and doctors in overseas facilities, primarily in France or Britain. Transport of military healthcare providers and soldiers was by sea, via military ships departing or arriving through the ports of New York City. Nurses in Europe worked at small military hospitals and camps where they provided care in collaboration with their peer military medics and surgeons. Conditions were often unanticipated and difficult. The wounded soldiers were carried by other soldiers from the trenches to an area safe from enemy fire where they could be provided basic first aid-type care and then transported a few miles away for more extensive treatments. At these evacuation hospitals, wounds were cared for and surgery was performed if necessary. Eventually, all wounded soldiers were taken to base hospitals, and depending on their personal circumstances, they were cared for prior to return to the trenches or they were stabilized and sent to stateside hospitals for further care.

Trench warfare was perfected as face-to-face combat decreased and offensive tactics were developed to avoid contact with artillery fire. Wounds were deeper and more extensive and involved multiple organs, and significant infections occurred from contact with the soil in trenches or on the battlefield. Iron shrapnel and steel bullets caused considerable soft tissue damage. "The wounds which [nurses would] be called upon to handle and dress [were] such that [they had] never imagined it possible for a human being to be so fearfully hurt and yet to be alive" (Kalisch & Kalisch, 2004, p. 211). Asepsis was difficult, and prevented wounds from being treated effectively; the use of strong antiseptics was not without damage to the already traumatized wounds. An invaluable method of cleansing was discovered by Alexis Carrel and Henry Dakin. It was a chlorine solution that was effective for infection without tissue damage; it eventually became known as Dakin's solution and is still in use today (Kalisch & Kalisch, 2004, p. 211).

Recruitment of nurses became a priority from 1917 to 1918, and the Nursing Committee and various civilian nursing schools solicited new students in a wartime crusade that organized resources to permit expanded education options. Campaign posters were developed in association with the Red Cross. Middle-class women as well as high school and college students were targeted for their interest in the vocation of nursing. Surveys assessed many aspects of nursing, from the objections and difficulties of nursing to the image of a nurse and the reasons one might desire to be a nurse. These campaigns changed the approach to nursing education during the next 2 decades and before the end of the war, led to the development of the Army School of Nursing and a change in the age requirement of an applicant, decreasing it to 21 years of age (Kalisch & Kalisch, 2004).

Nursing Workforce Issues

A T THE TURN OF THE CENTURY, females were granted the opportunity to participate in activities outside the home and family environment in ways never before available to them. Women were allowed admission into training schools, and eventually colleges, to train for a vocation other than that of motherhood and family or community service. With these newfound prospects for all women, there were some groups who were still excluded and discriminated against. Nursing was essentially a White female profession; Florence Nightingale (1867) believed "women, by nature, were more suited for organizing, performing, and supervising the nursing care ... to take all power over the nursing out of the hands of men and put it into the hands of one female trained head" (O'Lynn & Tranberger, 2007, p. 24). This sentiment excluded men from the profession since they were not admitted into hospital training schools and educational facilities where nurses were trained. From the mid-1800s until the early 1960s, males were somewhat invisible in nursing venues. Prior to the Nightingale era, men were commonly involved in care of the sick and injured as is evidenced from reports describing male nurses who were monks, knights, or medics in the military. There were many male nurses who served during the Civil and Spanish–American Wars, but when the battles ceased, society dictated that they return to the businesses and farms from whence they came. A small number of these male nurses remained in nursing service caring for mentally ill patients or working on male wards. An even smaller percentage of male nurses were actually freed slaves who continued to function as nurses primarily in the South until the 20th century, when females replaced them (Sabin, 1997).

With an increased need for nurses in hospitals and on the battlefield, the demand for them eventually exceeded their availability. With the military patients coming home from World War I with battle wounds and mustard gas burns, hospital facilities and staff were taxed to the limit. This created a shortage of physicians and nurses, especially in the civilian sector. The shortages were further confounded by the loss of nurses during the flu epidemic, as they, too, became infected and were thus unable to work due to illness and death. In the United States, the Red Cross recruited more volunteers to contribute to the new cause at home of fighting the influenza epidemic while still managing military patients abroad and on American soil. To respond with the fullest utilization of nurses, volunteers, and medical supplies, the Red Cross created a national committee on influenza. During the war, this committee encouraged employers to allow staff to volunteer one night in the hospital to assist the nurses who were unable to do all that was required of them. If an employee was willing to do that, employers were strongly encouraged to give the employee a half day off, which allowed the employee time to rest from that service. This strategy provided nonskilled assistants who could do duties that did not require a registered nurse's time and it enabled the trained nurses time to perform duties that only they could (Crosby, 1989).

In 1908, the National Association of Colored Graduate Nurses (NACGN) was formed in New York City by Martha Franklin, who felt that discrimination, unregulated professional standards, and lack of educational or leadership opportunities existed. The graduate nurses came together to create a more sympathetic understanding of discrimination, to promote better administrative and educational standards, to elicit cooperation, and finally to secure contacts with other nursing leaders. Franklin, along with Mary Mahoney, the first trained Black nurse in the United States, organized a convention the following year to address the concerns of Black nurses and to support them professionally. The organization promoted their interests into the late 1930s. In 1942, when the Army recruited 56 Black nurses into the Army Nurse Corps, the NACGN coordinated an increase in the number of Black nurses across the nation. A decade later, after affiliating with the National League for Nurses, the NACGN joined with the ANA to support integration and promote racial collaboration (Massey, 1933; New York Public Library, n.d.).

Dock, Sanger, Emma Goldman, and others were concerned about the effects that male dominance in the United States had on the nursing profession. They worried about paternalism in leadership and physician governance of nurses in a society that did not recognize women's equality or contributions.

> Women's equality was an issue for nurses ... there were women's issues in the profession ... in terms of educational reform, the ability to control one's own labor, and in equal pay for equal work ... Until we possess the ballot, we may get up in the morning to find that all we had gained had been taken from us. (Dock, 1907, p. 901)

She further encouraged nurses to become involved in the suffrage movement so that they would not be

> ... an inert mass of indifference ... the modern nursing movement is emphatically an outcome of the original and general woman movement ... nurses are no longer a dull, uneducated class, but an intelligent army of workers, capable of continuous progress, and titled to comprehend the idea of social responsibility. (Dock, 1907, p. 896)

Other workforce issues for nurses were related to labor concerns and management of the emerging profession. These included environmental conditions, governance of the profession by nurses rather than physicians, standard educational requirements, registration and licensure, and state regulation by a board of nurses. Of great concern was the number of hours nurses worked, since most nurses still worked many more than 40 hours per week and often longer than 10- to 12-hour shifts per day. Others worked split shifts, which did not allow for adequate rest, nutrition, exercise, or socialization. Military nurses and those who worked during the epidemic were especially prone to shifts that were not conducive to a normal daily routine.

Licensure and Regulation

Licensure and regulation of nurses became an issue in the early 1900s. Nurses gained more respect and autonomy, yet they were not totally supported by their peers—medical doctors. The public did not clearly understand the role of the nurse, nor did they know what the nurses' credentials really meant. During the 1893 World's Fair activities in Chicago, nursing superintendents from Canada and the United States met to discuss nursing issues of the time. They were determined to standardize nursing education so that curriculums were similar in all training schools. Initially, they formed a nursing organization called the American Society of Superintendents of Training Schools for Nurses of the United States and Canada (Andrist, Nicholas, & Wolf, 2006). Dock and Nutting were two members of this organization who helped determine educational standards during the early 1900s. This group, which eventually became known as the Superintendents Society, was renamed the National League for Nursing Education in 1912. Today this organization is known as the National League for Nursing, and it is still the governing body for determining the goals of education related to nursing curriculum; it has attempted to standardize all nursing programs through a process of accreditation.

A second organization, the Nurses' Associated Alumnae of the United States and Canada, was created to address legal concerns and regulation of nurses. This association was to be a companion group to the Superintendents Society organized at the World's Fair (Andrist, et al., 2006). This nursing society became recognized as the ANA in 1911, and was responsible at that time for establishing criteria related to scope of practice, licensure, and legislation of the nursing profession. The ANA has worked to promote the nursing profession by protecting nurses' rights, describing aspects of nursing practice, establishing guidelines for practice, promoting a positive nursing image, and eventually lobbying for both women's rights and nursing rights, which, during that era, were not really separate issues. The national organization (ANA) and the state affiliates continue to be effective today as they influence legal aspects of nursing, regulate practice nationally, and define practice roles.

These early organizations were established to advance the science and profession of nursing; however, because they ultimately had different perspectives, there was some separation of power, which resulted in problems related to promoting the profession effectively. As Ashley described, these issues remained as late as 1976:

> With the control of education in the hands of one organization and the control of practice in the hands of another, gaps in communication were inevitable. The lack of concerted action by both educators and practitioners created serious problems ... With this separation of functions, the foundation was laid for continuing lack of unity ... the conflicts and misunderstandings still exist today. (1976, p.96)

Nurses who received formal training along with their nurse supervisors soon began to concede the need for registration or certification indicating supervised training. One of the reasons for this was the rise of some training programs, including one published in the *New York Tribune*, which promised "You can become a trained nurse by study at home. Send ten cents for a handsome catalogue. Anyone, regardless of age or physical condition [can] become a trained nurse by a mere few months" (as cited in Kalisch & Kalisch, 2004, p. 178). The catalogue showed a nurse with the traditional uniform of a cap and an apron ready to take care of a patient. The nurse also wore her nurse's badge and was depicted with a spoon and medicine bottle indicting that she was trained and capable of appropriate patient care (Kalisch & Kalisch, 2004, p. 178). These training programs issued diplomas despite the fact that they lacked elements of training considered to be necessary for preparation.

Prior to 1900, nurses in New Zealand, Australia, and Great Britain initiated guidelines for practice and licensure. The first registered nurse was a female who served with the Maori people of New Zealand. In 1901, a group of nurses met in New York to discuss nursing issues, specifically those of educational preparation. These nurses were part of the newly created International Council of Nurses. A resolution was proposed during that meeting to initiate state nurse registrations by Bedford Fenwick, a nurse from Great Britain:

> Whereas at the present time there is no generally accepted term or standard of training nor system of education nor examination for nurses in any country ... nurses should be carefully educated in the important duties allotted to them; there is no method, except in South Africa, of enabling the public

to discriminate easily between trained nurses and ignorant persons who assume that title ... it is the duty of every country to work for suitable legislative enactment regulating education of nurses and protecting the interests of the public ... by securing State examinations and public registration with the proper penalties for enforcing the same ... (Fenwick, 1901, p. 330)

New York became the first state to establish a board of examiners specifically for nurses. The New York State Federation of Women's Clubs aided nurses in their quest for recognition and accreditation standards along with other social and political concerns of the day, including women's suffrage. During the next several years, many other states attempted to initiate legislation regulating nurses. North Carolina proposed legislation in 1903 for mandatory educational requirements and regulation of nurses, but there was "strong opposition by the lobby of the state medical society" (Kalisch & Kalisch, 2004, p. 179) such that the bill was altered to include only certification by exam. If an applicant could pass the examination, education in a nurse training program did not need to be documented. The state board of examiners, according to the legislation, would include three physicians and two nurses (Kalisch & Kalisch, 2004). This allowed the medical community to be involved in regulating nursing practice, which has continued to be problematic into the 21st century.

Nursing Research

CONCERNS OVER EDUCATIONAL STANDARDS and funding prevailed during the early 1900s not only for nursing but for medicine in general. In 1910, Abraham Flexner prepared a report funded by the Carnegie Foundation discussing inadequacies in medical education. The following year, Nutting and some others decided at the convention of the American Society of Superintendents of Training Schools for Nurses that a similar study should be undertaken to assess educational standards, to document areas of concern, and to describe possible solutions. Much of what has been described in this chapter related to education, licensure, regulation, and practice were defined or reinforced as a result of this study. Even though nurse advocates did not conduct research in the same manner that we do today, they changed nursing for the better through their activities.

Many organizers of nursing groups, nurse superintendents, and nurses of that era contributed to research as they reported what they did and their results. They intervened in the community with services that changed mortality and morbidity. Frontier nurses and rural nurses decreased infant mortality, postpartum infections, and complications. All community and public health nurses helped to eliminate trachoma, tuberculosis, and common infectious diseases as they understood more about sanitation and contagious diseases. School nurses controlled skin infections, lice, and other common childhood ailments and increased opportunities for children to attend school. Other public health nurses dealt with women and children's health concerns and documented positive outcomes as they did. Even controversial ideas, such as Sanger's birth control and sex education programs, enabled nurses to serve the community in ways that decreased suffering while eliminating ignorance. Remember, public health nurses were instrumental in establishing criteria and standards of practice, including standing orders for which they were recognized and eventually sanctioned when the Metropolitan Life Insurance Company advocated for them by reimbursing for their services, which were of great worth to the community.

Summary

NURSING DURING THE EARLIEST DECADES of the 20th century changed dramatically from the vocation that it had been during the later part of the 19th century. Many aspects of nursing today were influenced by events that promoted new opportunities and roles for women during this time, and by the observations and recommendations of nurses who worked relentlessly to promote nursing as an honest and worthy endeavor. Medical care changed dramatically across this era as a result of many medical advances, a world war, two epidemics, changes in nursing education, the creation of nursing organizations, the expansion of public health or community nursing, the promotion of women's rights nationally, the acknowledgement of women's health concerns, greater recognition of childhood issues, and promotion of hospitals as a better way to provide medical care. Many of the principal nurses of these decades influenced nursing while acting as political and social reformers as well. As the public's perception of nursing and the importance of nurses' roles in the lives of the American people became evident, nurses gained a more positive image and nursing was perceived as a profession rather than a job.

◆ IDEAS FOR FURTHER EXPLORATION

1. Investigate and discover more about World War I and the effects it had on nurses, who were predominantly women.
2. Assess how women's suffrage affected nursing opportunities and education. Who were some of the nurses in the United States who supported it and eventually promoted changes for the health of women and children in all areas of the country? What programs did they initiate and support?
3. During the first 20 years of the 20th century, what scientific advances and discoveries related to health care impacted nursing care? Research historical records to learn about discoveries not discussed in this text.
4. How did the influenza epidemic change health care and orientation to infectious diseases?

◆ DISCUSSION QUESTIONS: APPLICATION TO CURRENT PRACTICE

1. Changes in licensure and education occurred in nursing during the early 1900s. How did/do those recommendations affect nurses today? Does the profession still have these same concerns? Why or why not?
2. Identify and describe nursing organizations that were instituted in the early 1900s. Are they still in existence today, and what, if any, influence do they have on the various aspects of nursing practice in the 21st century?
3. Industrialization and technology influenced healthcare options around 1900. Identify how community health changed the world of health care. What advances occurred and how did hospitals and insurance programs fit into the management of health? Give specific examples of then and now scenarios in the healthcare industry.

⁕ MeSH SEARCH TERMS

World War I

Other useful non-MesH terms:

Army Nurse Corps

Navy Nurse Corps

Spanish flu

National Association of Colored Graduate Nurses

National League for Nursing Education

American Nurses Association

Henry Street Settlement

Adelaide Nutting

Lillian Wald

Lavinia Dock

Margaret Sanger

⁕ SUGGESTED READING

Budreau, L. M., & Prior, R. M. (2008). *Answering the call: The U.S. Army Nurse Corps, 1917–1919: A commemorative tribute to military nursing in World War I.* Washington, DC: Office of the Surgeon General, Borden Institute, Walter Reed Army Medical Center.

Marshall, H. E. (1972). *Mary Adelaide Nutting, pioneer of modern nursing.* Baltimore: Johns Hopkins University Press.

Nutting, M. A. & Dock, L. L . (1907–1912). *A history of nursing: The evolution of nursing systems from the earliest times to the foundation of the first English and American training schools for nurses.* New York: G.P. Putnam's Sons.

Wald, L. D. (1915). *The house on Henry Street.* New York: Henry Holt and Company.

⁕ REFERENCES

American Academy of Medicine. (1913). *Medical problems of immigration, being the papers and their discussion presented at the XXXVII annual meeting of the American Academy of Medicine, held at Atlantic City, June 1, 1912.* Easton, PA: American Academy of Medicine Press.

Andrist, L. C., Nicholas, P. K., & Wolf, K. A. (Eds.). (2006). *A history of nursing ideas.* Sudbury, MA: Jones and Bartlett.

Ashley, J. A. (1976). *Hospitals, paternalism, and the role of the nurse.* New York: Teachers College Press.

Barry, J. M. (2005). *The great influenza: The epic story of the deadliest plague in history.* New York: Penguin Books.

Billings, M. (2005). *The influenza pandemic of 1918.* Retrieved August 2, 2008, from http://virus.stanford.edu/uda/

Brinkley, A. (2003). *American history: A survey* (11th ed.). New York: McGraw-Hill.

Crosby, A. W. (1989). *America's forgotten pandemic: The influenza of 1918.* Cambridge, MA: Cambridge University Press.

Dock, L. L. (1907). Some urgent claims. *American Journal of Nursing, 7*(10), 895–901.

Donahue, M. P. (1996). *Nursing: The finest art* (2nd ed.). St. Louis, MO: Mosby.

Fenwick, B. (1901). International unity on state registration [Editorial]. *The Nursing Record and Hospital World, 27*(708), 329–330.

Foley, E. L. (1913). Departments of visiting nursing and social welfare. *American Journal of Nursing. 13*(6), 451–455.

Goodrich, A. W. (1932). *The school of nursing and the future: Proceedings of the thirty-eighth annual convention of the National League of Nursing Education.* New York: National League of Nursing Education, National Headquarters.

Houweling, L. (2004). Image, function, and style: A history of the nursing uniform. *American Journal of Nursing, 104*(4), 40–48.

Jewish Women's Archive. (2008a). *Exhibit: Women of Valor—Lillian Wald; Federal Children's Bureau.* Retrieved July 31, 2008, from http://jwa.org/exhibits/wov/wald/lw14.html

Jewish Women's Archive. (2008b). *Exhibit: Women of Valor—Lillian Wald; Henry Street Settlement.* Retrieved July 31, 2008 from http://jwa.org/exhibits/wov/wald/lw4.html

Kalisch, P. A., & Kalisch, B. J. (2004). *American nursing: A history* (4th ed.). Philadelphia: Lippincott, Williams, and Wilkins.

Kerber, L. K. & De Hart, J. S. (1995). *Women's America: Refocusing the past* (4th ed.). New York: Oxford University Press.

Massey, G. E. (1933). The National Association of Graduate Colored Nurses. *The American Journal of Nursing, 33*(6), 534–536.

Mosby, Inc. (2000). *Nursing reflections: A century of caring.* St. Louis, MO: Mosby.

The need of a standard uniform. (1916). *American Journal of Nursing, 16*(10), 966–967.

New York Public Library. (n.d.). *Inventory of the National Association of Colored Graduate Nurses Records 1908–1951: Sc Micro 7004 (Sc MG 16).* Retrieved August 31, 2008, from: http://www.nypl.org/research/manuscripts/scm/scmnacgn.xml

O'Lynn, C. E., & Tranbarger, R. E. (Eds.). (2007). *Men in nursing: History, challenges, and opportunities.* New York: Springer.

Rinehart, M. R. (1931). *My story.* New York: Farrar & Rinehart.

Sabin, L. E. (1997). Unheralded nurses; Male care givers in the nineteenth-century South. *Nursing History Review, 5,* 131–148.

Sanger, M. (1922). *The pivot of civilization.* New York: Brentano's Publishers.

Stewart, I. M. (1943). *The education of nurses: Historical foundations and modern trends.* New York: The Macmillan Co.

United States Public Health Service. (1939). Bubonic plague outbreak in San Francisco—Year 1900. *California and Western Medicine, 50*(2), 121–123. Retrieved June 23, 2008, from http://www.pubmedcentral.nih.gov/articlerender.fcgi?artid=1659815

CHAPTER 6

Nursing in the United States From the 1920s to the Early 1940s

1925–1940
- Public health nursing expanded
- Trachoma eradicated
- Sanitation practices reduce infectious diseases

1921
Margaret Sanger establishes American Birth Control League in New York

1925
Kentucky Frontier Nurses Services initiated

1927
Charles Lindbergh flies across the Atlantic Ocean

1929
- Stock market crash begins the Great Depression
- Alexander Fleming describes penicillin

1920	1921	1922	1923	1924	1925	1926	1927	1928	1929

1920
- 19th Amendment passed, enables women to vote
- Prohibition enforced

1922
- Insulin discovered
- Sigma Theta Tau formed

1928
First portable electrocardiogram used

1920–1935 Nursing schools adopt standardized curriculum

EDUCATION RATHER THAN TRAINING FOR NURSES

Deborah M. Judd

1935
- Sulfonomides identified
- Social Security Act

| 1930 | 1931 | 1932 | 1933 | 1934 | 1935 | 1936 | 1937 | 1938 | 1939 | 1940 |

1932
Low point of the Depression

1938
- The atom is split
- Fair Labor Act creates minimum wage

Early 1940s
National League for Nursing proposes national test for nurses

1930s
- Association of Collegiate Schools of Nursing is formed
- Midwifery programs organized, training is standardized
- Educational reform leads to the grading of nursing schools
- Licensure exams refined

1932–1933 Nursing schools adopt standardized curriculum

1940
National Council for War Service founded to coordinate nursing services during wartime

OUR NURSING HERITAGE: KEY PEOPLE

Florence G. Blake	Established criteria for pediatric nursing curriculums Developed standards for pediatric clinical experiences
Mary Breckinridge	Founded the Frontier Nursing Service, the first rural healthcare system Organized the Frontier Nursing Service School
Mary Elizabeth Carnegie	Instituted the Black nursing program in Virginia Served on the American Nurses Association's Minority Fellowship Program Advisory Committee Authored *The Path We Tread: Blacks in Nursing Worldwide, 1854-1994*
Signe Skott Cooper	Encouraged continuing education for all nurses Developed a telephone conferencing course in the mid 1960s
Agnes K. Ohlson	Contributed to the ANA's discussion of state testing standards Worked to develop the first national standardized nursing test, eventually known as the State Board Test Pool Examination
Margaret Sanger	Opened the first U.S. birth control clinic Founded the American Birth Control League and Planned Parenthood Supported the women's suffrage movement Cared for the public living in poverty
Isabel M. Stewart	Promoted nursing curriculum development Continued the work of Adelaide Nutting Wrote a nursing history book with her peer Lavinia Dock
Shirley Carew Titus	Promoted nursing's responsibility to improve economic security through the ANA Inspired the 1946 ANA convention platform supporting collective bargaining Authored *Economic Security Is Not Too Much to Ask*
Susie Walking Bear Yellowtail	Native American visiting nurse who assessed health and health care on Native American reservations Promoted government aid to fund tribal nurses

Sociopolitical Climate

WITH THE END OF WORLD WAR I, the United States experienced relief, in part, due to the relatively short encounter and the somewhat low combat causalities; over half of the 112,000 who lost their lives during the war succumbed to influenza or other diseases rather than dying in combat. The war itself provided an economic boost to the nation as industry and technology increased, initiating an era of prosperity and ease for many. Minority populations had opportunities to work in advancing industries causing population shifts among the Asians, African Americans, and Mexicans of the nation. Dramatic changes occurred in cities as thousands of African Americans migrated from the South into areas of the North where industry had boomed. Similar situations appeared in the West as Asians and Mexicans traveled to agricultural centers in California and Texas or to cities such as the industrial city, San Francisco.

> The 'Great Migration' was a result of both a push and a pull. The push was the poverty, indebtedness, racism, and violence most blacks experienced in the South. The pull was the prospect of factory jobs and opportunity ... communities where [they] could enjoy more freedom and autonomy. (Brinkley, 2003, p. 631)

With this change in community dynamics, distress occurred as Whites and minorities adjusted to living together in new ways.

The United States emerged a world power and became a beacon for world unity. In reality, there was only discouragement and frustration by the end of this era since "the war to end all wars ... the war to make the world safe for democracy, became neither of those. Instead, it led to twenty years of international instability and another conflict" (Brinkley, 2003, p. 621), that being World War II. In the early 1940s, the United States entered this war defensively. As Britain and France tried to make peace with Germany, the United States attempted to promote principles that would lead to improved international conduct—open agreements rather than secret treaties, arms reductions, unrestricted seafaring, free exchanges (trade), and collaborative arbitration related to colonial issues. Country boundaries and disputes over control affected the nation's relationship with Russia well into the 1930s, while the Allies formed more permanent alliances as a result of the formation of the League of Nations (Brinkley, 2003).

The population of the United States exceeded 100 million during 1920 as the nation faced a number of social and political issues related to immigrants, women, children, the ever-expanding economy, and a perceived era of affluence (Mosby, Inc., 2000). The Roaring Twenties was a time of gaiety and changes in social norms associated with many new freedoms for women and their ability to participate more readily in activities outside the home.

> Some women concluded in the 'New Era' that it was no longer necessary to maintain rigid "respectability". They could smoke, drink, dance, and wear seductive clothes and makeup . . . they strive for physical and emotional fulfillment, a release from repression and inhibition. (Brinkley, 2003, pp. 658–659)

Although many women were intrigued with the new image of women and the opportunities of leisure and employment it implied, most women still married and were in a satisfied relationship. Those who pursued a career generally chose between work and a family.

Conservatives believed that Prohibition would decrease activities that were less than desirable in the nation, yet in retrospect, it is clear that there were considerable increases in criminal activities as underground liquor production and speakeasy establishments emerged in most communities. Many became rich selling the banned liquor, which became readily available to almost anyone who desired it, even in smaller communities. As significant resources were expended by the federal government in an effort to enforce the law, those who so vigorously supported Prohibition and the Eighteenth Amendment were no longer as committed to the cause. Over time the graft, the gangs, the deaths, and the corruption led many to reconsider the legislation. It wasn't until 1933 that Prohibition was finally repealed and the "empire of over 1000 gunmen organized by Al Capone" and others was thwarted (Brinkley, 2003, p. 665).

Unions flourished until the beginning of the 1920s, when capitalistic democracy became popular, resulting in a movement entitled the American Plan. This was intended to alleviate unions and set up open shops where the workers could decide if they would join the union or not. The Supreme Court eventually intervened and prohibited picketing and strikes in an effort to control abusive union powers. Economic growth increased substantially, and by 1929 it was unimaginable to think that in one day all that could change. The stock market crash in 1929 ushered in the Great Depression, and with it much suffering and loss (Brinkley, 2003).

Despite prosperity prior to the Great Depression, many "remained outside the reach of the new affluent consumer culture" (Brinkley, 2002, pp. 650–651) and disparity became an issue in many urban and agricultural areas of the nation. New technology and sophisticated engines and machinery replaced human service, decreasing the number of workers required to perform some jobs. Additionally, service careers that required advanced education were expanding, creating gaps in eligibility and obtainable employment. Education in general became important to those who could afford it or who had access to it. From 1920 to 1930, there was a threefold increase in the number of students enrolled in either a college or a university and high school attendance nationally doubled during that same period of time (Brinkley, 2003).

Women's suffrage created an environment for freedoms never before imagined by women, but it also promoted White supremacy, creating further ethnic and racial tensions. During 1921, Congress enacted legislation limiting immigration and establishing annual quotas. In the South and in northern cities where African Americans had migrated for employment, the rise of the Ku Klux Klan led to clashes and the idea of ethnic cleansing during the 1920s. However, "[w]hat the 'Klan' feared was not simply foreign or racially impure groups," but any group that challenged traditional values and morals (Brinkley, 2003, p. 667). The Ku Klux Klan all but disappeared in the North by the early 1930s, yet in the South after World War II, it revitalized and was problematic as attempts to end segregation ensued from 1940 to 1970. Racial issues escalated as the 20th century progressed, and eventually the nation had to make choices to eliminate segregation through legislation and minority activists.

The Image of Nursing

Nurses continued to wear modest dresses, caps, and aprons in the hospital setting, while their counterparts in community or rural areas of the nation wore modest dresses, frequently with white collars and cuffs on their blue uniforms and hats that reflected some of the style of the flappers with a cape or cloak. Dresses were calf length and sleeves were sometimes three-quarter length or to the elbow. The bodices were not as form fitting as

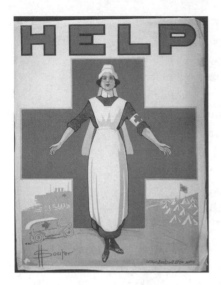

"Help" poster by D.H. Souter used to recruit nurses in World War I shows nurse in uniform

they had been at the turn of the century, allowing for more flexible movement when caring for the patient. Uniforms were still associated with the type of service the nurse provided, so a hospital uniform was different from a community nurse uniform, and of course the military nurse uniform was unique. Military nurses not only had uniforms for patient care, but they also had military uniforms for parades and other public appearances.

The school or hospital where nurses were trained or employed still determined what type of cap or dress was worn by their nurses. White or very light colored fabrics were becoming the standard for many hospital nurses; however, it wasn't until the 1940s that the traditional white uniform became nearly universal. Many nurses felt that the uniform was a distinguishing feature of the profession, and they did not want others to have a uniform that resembled theirs. A selected group of nurses encouraged a different style of dress since they determined maids or waitresses wore a similar uniform with an apron (Houweling, 2004). Other nurses and students felt that as they gained more autonomy, a standard uniform determined by the organization or school remained an aspect of continued control over the profession. The black bag in which the community nurse carried her supplies was still a symbol of her ability and training to care for those in the community adequately.

The Education of Nurses

WITH MORE FOCUS ON THEORY and new supplementary courses in the curriculum, nurses were better prepared to care for those in the hospital or the community. Preliminary courses were required for most nursing students as they were taught to understand even the simplest procedures before actually performing them on a patient, a precursor to what is now the clinical skills lab educational experience. "Advocates of higher education believed that the better a woman understands her work, the better she will do it ... good bedside nursing demands specialized scientific training" (Goodnow, 1943, p. 221). By 1910, about 100 hospital schools were providing preparatory classes along with practical training, which included scientific foundations of fundamental care to support bedside nursing.

One characteristic of a profession is specific and ample training; in order to meet this professional requirement, student nurses were required to have a high school diploma with satisfactory grades and complete very specific educational requisites. Screening tests were often used to assess "scholastic and mechanical aptitude, ability in reading and arithmetic, vocabulary, and sometimes personality traits" (Goodnow, 1943, pp. 221–222) prior to acceptance into the discipline. Students were expected to complete coursework in medical, surgical, and obstetrical patient care. Psychiatry rotations became mandatory by the 1940s. Some hospitals lacked pediatric or obstetrical patients in the early 1920s, making their schools ineligible for accreditation. All accredited schools provided rotations where students cared for men, women, and children (Goodnow, 1943). Male nursing students encountered difficulties, since in most hospitals they were not allowed to care for obstetrical patients. In Illinois, the Alexian Brothers' Schools of Nursing for male students were accredited in 1925 and male students were given the option of substituting urology for obstetrics, and when they took their written exam they were given an option to replace the obstetrics portion with urology. Until 1958, this substitution was an acceptable alternative; however, after that time, all nursing students were required to rotate through obstetrical wards (O'Lynn & Tranbarger, 2007).

Nursing schools were no longer independent and isolated when it came to development of their educational standards and goals. As universal curriculum recommendations were initiated and eventually encouraged as mandatory, state boards of nursing attempted to promote them in their respective states. During that era, the National League for Nursing established criteria for accreditation and published a list of schools that met the requirements. With the formation of state nursing boards after 1905, legal aspects of practice were determined. The first state to describe exactly what was to be taught and when it should be taught was New York. Shortly thereafter, the American Nurses Association suggested a standard curriculum intended to promote unity among nursing schools nationally. The suggested guidelines were clarified during the 1920s, and many schools of nursing adopted them by 1935 as they tried to improve the quality and content of nursing programs. The effort to develop better nursing ensured definite improvements, both at that time and well into the future. Nursing leaders promoted education rather than training in order for students to acquire knowledge which would guide them and the profession.

Affiliations among nursing schools and hospital facilities ensued as collaborative relationships developed, nurse education was redefined, and schools were connected to universities or colleges rather than just hospitals. The Rockefeller Foundation surveyed typical nursing schools and suggested that a basic nursing course should be 28 months for bedside nursing, 8–9 months for nurse's aid training, and that any nurse working in public health, executive health, or teaching positions should have a postgraduate course (postgraduate course at that time referred to classes after the basic education). Finally, they proposed that endowments should be made available to nursing schools in order to promote educational opportunities for those who otherwise did not have them (Goodnow, 1943).

Schools of nursing adopted the belief that better schools of nursing focused education on the clinical experiences and theory and not on the idea that the service students provided in the hospital would allow them to learn how to be nurses. Universities, colleges, and hospital programs worked independently using proposed guidelines to develop educational programs that would allow for a student nurse to leave the program with an academic diploma. These new graduate nurses could then take a licensure exam that would allow them to practice legally with their new credentials. The Associate Degree in Nursing was one of the results of these innovative programs; in later years there was controversy associated with this community college degree, as well as the hospital diploma program.

Advances in Nursing Practice

DURING THE LATER PART OF the 1920s, community nursing became recognized as a very valuable resource for overall public health. Since many immigrants relied on self-medication and traditional cures, they did not seek medical care, nor were they likely to go to the hospital.

> For every ill there is a sure cure provided in print ... *Dr This* is as confident of removing your cancer without the use of the knife, as *Dr That* is of

eradicating your consumption by his marvelous new discovery ... The more deadly the disease, the more blatantly certain is the quack that he alone can save you ... (Kalisch & Kalisch, 2004, p. 255)

Most professional health care was provided in the home during this period of nursing history. When the scope of public health nursing was defined during the 1920s, the primary duty of the nurse was patient advisor; advisors shared best techniques and knowledge about illness and health. As these services were recognized and considered successful, the U.S. Health Department promoted funding and encouraged community participation in these programs. However, only 41% of cities with a population over 10,000 had community nurses who worked full time; communities funded on average $14.00 per individual for education while only spending 91¢ per person on health promotion and disease management. According to Kalisch & Kalisch (2004), they dealt "firsthand with communicable diseases, inspecting milk and other food, maintaining a pure water supply, conducting clinics, providing nursing service, and reaching the people with health instruction" (p. 252).

With advancements in science and better understanding of medications, sanitation, and body processes, new knowledge was being transferred to

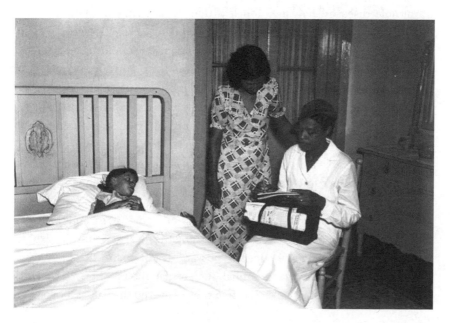

Nurse making a house call, New Orleans, Louisisana

individuals and their families through public health nurses. They promoted new health practices. For example, visiting nurses taught mothers that syrups distributed by various traveling healers to be used for a colicky baby often contained morphine in the solution and might cause morphine poisoning, respiratory distress, and even death. Frontier nurses encouraged well-child checks for infants and preschoolers while providing immunizations for typhoid, diphtheria, and smallpox, which reduced mortality rates dramatically. They organized health demonstrations in many communities. Nurse-midwives with specific training participated during deliveries in rural areas, decreasing infant mortality during the first year by more than one third and stillbirths by about the same percentage (Kalisch & Kalisch, 2004).

Throughout the country, health demonstrations became popular to promote certain aspects of health, the benefit of public health services, and to enlighten people on the programs and care available to them individually. From 1920 to 1923, diagnostic standards improved and disease mortality decreased by about two thirds as public health nurses and local physicians worked together to screen, educate, and treat. Most people with advanced disease still were hospitalized in a sanitarium where hospital nurses and aides cared for them (Kalisch & Kalisch, 2004).

Still, most health concerns had to do with lack of education about communicable diseases, hygiene, and less than ideal living conditions. Many did not know when, how, or why to seek medical care. Diseases such as dysentery, severe shortness of breath or pneumonias, and fevers that did not resolve were reasons people might seek medical care, but infections like measles, mumps, sore throats, colds, and coughs were often treated at home without any medical intervention. Pregnancy and birth were normal aspects of life, as were death and dying, so it was not recognized that seeking medical or nursing care could be of benefit in such circumstances. Mary Breckinridge recognized a need for prenatal, natal, and postnatal care. In the mid 1920s, she was instrumental in organizing the Frontier Nursing program in Kentucky.

She found that most lay midwives could not read or write and that none had formal training; midwifery was something they learned through experience, and there were many superstitions and traditions in their practices. In some cases midwives were familial, such as daughters following mothers who had provided such a service. Often they delivered the babies alone, with the help of a friend or family member. If complications arose, most times there was no physician called since that might demean their competency. These lay midwives would try the following:

> ... to stop hemorrhage by repeating certain Bible verses or by making tea from black gum bark from the north side of the tree mixed with the bark of sweet apple tree from the south side of the tree. Soot was used extensively as a medication ... (Kalisch & Kalisch, 2004, p. 258)

One strategy to prevent birthing problems was the use of an axe placed under the bed with the blade up during the delivery.

After receiving formal training in England, Breckinridge organized a group of frontier nurses in Kentucky who were designated to serve in a specific area monitoring public health and managing pregnancies. These nurses would travel by foot or on horseback, answering calls while caring for patients who were pregnant. They made home visits twice a month for seven months, and then weekly until delivery. Infants were followed twice a month during their first year of life and then each quarter until age 5 or 6. As part of these frontier services, a small hospital was organized and managed by two nurses and a doctor. Patients could receive care either at home or in the hospital. Normal pregnancies and deliveries were the responsibility of the nurse-midwives; anyone with complications was referred to the doctor. Once they delivered, the nurse-midwives resumed care of the mother and her children. All services were made available for a yearly fee of $1.00, and if patients could not pay, services still might be granted. In essence, this was one of the first managed healthcare groups (Dublin, 1932).

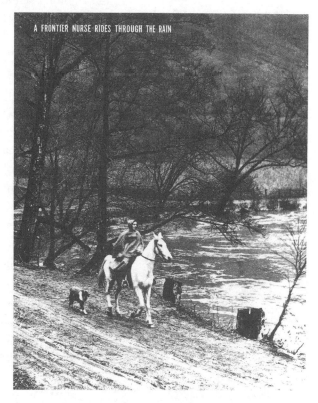

A FRONTIER NURSE RIDES THROUGH THE RAIN

"A frontier nurse rides through the rain," by Marvin Breckinridge Patterson

The frontier nurses received guidance from nurses trained in England or Scotland prior to the mid-1930s, when midwifery programs were organized and training was standardized to a certain extent in the United States. Through the interventions of these competent nurses, antenatal troubles, complications at delivery, stillbirths, maternal deaths, and problems during the postpartum period decreased by a third. The Metropolitan Life Insurance Company promoted and supported an insurance health program that was based on the successful endeavors of these dedicated frontier nurses starting in the early 1930s (Dublin, 1932).

The U.S. Public Health Services instituted a number of other healthcare programs from 1920 to 1940. Trachoma, an infection of the eye which started in the conjunctiva, eventually causing deformity and blindness, was prevalent in certain regions of the country and reached epidemic proportions in many communities and on Indian reservations among schoolchildren. A substantial part of the U.S. Public Health Service budget was earmarked to fight this disease. Numerous trachoma surveys revealed the presence of a trachoma belt across the middle of the United States, and the prevalence of trachoma reached as high as 50–90% among schoolchildren on some Indian reservations. Crowding, poverty, and lack of clean water and hygiene were identified as risk factors for trachoma. Measures taken to combat the disease included isolation schools for infected children, special government trachoma hospitals and field clinics, screening of immigrants entering the United States, improvements in hygiene and sanitation, and antibiotic therapy. The Indian Health Service attempted radical eyelid surgery because the problem was so widespread on the reservations; it reported disastrous consequences.

Although largely considered a problem of developing countries today, trachoma was extremely common in parts of the United States at this time and accounted for a large proportion of blindness. Rural nurses in Virginia, West Virginia, Missouri, Kentucky, Arkansas,

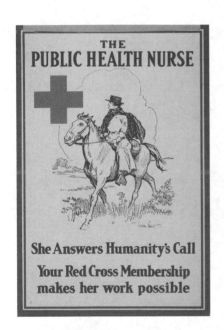

"The Public Health Nurse: She Answers Humanity's Call; Your Red Cross Membership makes her work possible," poster by Gordon Grant

and Tennessee became involved in the trachoma program designed to control and eventually eliminate the disease. Nurses would make rounds and identify those with the disease, and then isolate them in a clinic or specialty hospital ward where treatment commenced. Once a case of trachoma was identified, treatment included multiple eye irrigations each day, instillation of silver nitrate and possibly atropine, and education on hygiene. Although the source of the infection was not identified at the time, crowding and poor sanitation were felt to be factors. Eventually it was discovered that a fly was responsible for the spread of the disease from one individual's eye to another. Nurses in these communities did great work as they eliminated blindness through new knowledge and techniques (Allen & Semba, 2002). Prevalence surveys showed a clear decline in trachoma in the United States during the 20th century because of these interventions and programs (Allen & Semba, 2002).

Margaret Sanger continued her work with women in the community and eventually wrote *The Pivot of Civilization*, which promoted full reproductive freedom for women (Sanger, 1922). In the early 1920s, Sanger established the Birth Control League in New York City. Later she founded the National Committee on Federal Legislation for Birth Control. Her Birth Control League was the predecessor of Planned Parenthood, an organization which still is in existence today, providing women's healthcare services. For decades there was opposition to her work, yet she persevered in her cause until her death in 1966. During the year prior to her death, the Supreme Court ruled that married couples did have the right to decide upon birth control in their marriage.

The word *hygiene* comes from Hygeia, one of the daughters of the Greek god Aesculapius. Advancing knowledge about germ theories from the mid-1800s to the mid-1900s focused medical evolution on "hygiene and sanitation ... the forefront of the struggle against illness and disease". Faria (2002) further emphasizes that these two focus areas "resulted in unprecedented longevity, concomitant with markedly improved quality of life in the last century and a half," referring to the era from 1850 to 2000 (Faria, 2002, pp. 122–123). Childbirth fever was almost eradicated because obstetricians and nurses washed their hands regularly between patient deliveries. In the 1930s, the use of antibiotics and improved standards of cleanliness improved life expectancy, and many infectious diseases were controlled.

During the 1920s, vaccines for diphtheria, pertussis, tuberculosis, and tetanus were introduced. The result was an increase in life expectancy from 59.7 years to 74.9 years over the next 30 years (Faria, 2002, pp. 122–123).

War and Its Effects on Nursing

AFTER WORLD WAR I, MILITARY nurses returned to civilian hospitals and community nursing service for the most part, while some continued to care for military personnel and soldiers who still needed medical care as a result of their involvement in the war. The army had been the largest employer of nurses during the war, but that did not continue through the years of peace, social reform, and financial distress that followed. With educational recommendations and modifications occurring as the next war became imminent, military leaders felt the need to be proactive in preparing for the anticipated need for nursing services.

In 1936, Joseph Stalin began a campaign to eliminate enemies within the Soviet Republic, and millions were either imprisoned or killed before World War II commenced on European soil when German soldiers invaded Poland. Although the United States was not involved in war efforts until 1941, a National Council for War Service was founded in 1940 to coordinate nursing service during war. This organization was to determine criteria for unification for all nurses, from recruitment and training to actual care given in a military situation. Army and navy nurses were trained in accordance with protocols established during World War I, and eventually according to the curriculum developed at the Army School of Nursing, which was determined in part by existing national nursing associations.

Nursing Workforce Issues

DURING THE 1920S, THE MAJORITY of registered nurses worked as private duty nurses, but with the stock market crash in 1929, patients and families could no longer pay for private duty services. About 20% of the labor force lost their jobs during this recession, and even nurses in the hospital were concerned about continued employment. Despite the overall unemployment trends, women continued to participate in work activities outside the home. The Great Depression caused major personal financial challenges for almost all citizens, and many lost property and jobs. As the recession years continued, private duty nurses were affected the most, yet all nurses found it difficult to find work or even keep the jobs they had. Substantial unemployment created concerns for graduate nurses, and the *American Journal of Nursing* posted bulletins such as: "Nurses who are contemplating coming to New York to work are advised not to do so as there is not enough work for nurses already here" (Kalisch & Kalisch, 2004, p. 271). Another message read: "To nurses contemplating coming to Miami.... There are several hundred nurses out of employment ... there is less work here than there has been at any time in the past eleven years" (Kalisch & Kalisch, 2004, p. 271). A tax was sometimes charged in addition to the registration fees of the state in order for nurses to be able to practice in the state.

The Public Health Services offered nurses a reduced salary, which allowed for some of them to continue working to care for the public and have a limited income while it helped the government deal with budget concerns. Another innovative measure tried by hospitals was the employment of graduate nurses for room, board, and laundry instead of direct wages. Kalisch and Kalisch indicate that there were concerns that those nurses who were willing to work under such circumstances "gave inferior service and often were not even worth their food and lodging" and that the hospital budget would be adversely affected since "the expense of the additional board and laundry [of] these extra graduate nurses" would not be worth it (2004, p. 273). Others felt that in such a circumstance the hospital actually "should not take advantage of the unemployed nurse ... a most unfair advantage of the graduate nurse's helpless situation" (Kalisch & Kalisch, 2004, p. 273). Thus, the Depression forced nurses into the hospital as they left behind community nursing, a service that focused on the prevention of unnecessary deaths, the elimination of blindness, the introduction of new ideas about disease causes, and ways to decrease the spread of those diseases, enhance nutrition, and improve sanitation (Andrist, Nicholas, & Wolf, 2006, p. 394). This was the impetus needed to promote hospital nursing and the notion that nurses cared for patients in the acute care setting very effectively.

Community and rural nurses spent their time caring for patients individually, and though some were private duty nurses, most were home visiting nurses who administered care to specific individuals or families. As they spent time in patient's homes, they would instruct them on basic treatments for common ailments such as fevers or colds. They also taught patients and families about food preparation, sanitation, infant concerns and problems, childhood illness, nutrition, and childbirth. Traveling salesmen and self-proclaimed healers were less prevalent than they were 20 years earlier, yet community nurses still spent considerable time trying to banish unsafe practices while promoting new knowledge to those who still believed in traditional ideas and cures. Nurses who worked in these communities faced challenges as they tried to introduce new ideas about health and wellness to individuals and families who did not always want to change.

With the advent of educational reforms, there were questions about how to proceed. In 1925, the American Nurses Association sponsored a 5-year study to assess conditions of nursing schools in 10 states. The Committee on the Grading of Nursing Schools included nurses, doctors, and lay people. The committee encouraged nursing schools to

> cherish your apprentice system ... it is absolutely unique in the actual living situation—what patients need, where they need it, and when they need it. [Do not] attempt to make nursing schools into copies of other schools, there is much in the existing system of nursing education which is admirable and meticulous. (Goodnow, 1943, p. 226)

Routine student nursing labor had become the norm for most hospital programs; debate arose among nursing leaders who felt that the older system of apprenticeship should be replaced with "the newer method of giving scientific approach to the work ... We have [to] make a distinction between a nurse's training and an education in nursing" (Goodnow, 1943, p. 219).

As the dialogue about training versus education continued, there was the need for direction on preparation of nurses. It took some time for hospitals to relinquish their control of the nurse's education and for staff nurses to accept graduate nurses. Recommendations that changed nursing education could be summarized as follows:

1. Training was to be for the student's benefit and not for the hospital's benefit.

2. Schools should take fewer students in order to train them more effectively.

3. Each school should be evaluated for its efficiency in its community.

4. National standards should focus on education and specific aspects of care.

5. Schools should strive for accreditation in order to regulate education.

6. Nursing students should abide by the standard 40-hour workweek.

These guidelines established theoretical and clinical curriculums and programs in colleges and universities and forced hospital schools to change the way they trained nurses (Hall, 1929).

Opportunity greeted one group, while exclusion and discrimination greeted all of the others. Nursing remained essentially a female profession, and despite the need for both military and civilian nurses, males and Black nurses were not accepted into military nurse corps. Educational opportunities were very limited for them in hospital, university, or college-affiliated training schools. In the mid-1920s, Black hospitals emerged in the South along with more than 25 new nursing schools for Black students. For the next 20–30 years, segregation would affect healthcare options and nursing school applicants. In Harlem, two new nursing schools were organized to serve the Black community. With an increase in the number of facilities for Blacks, segregation was actually promoted and integration was sacrificed as further isolation resulted. The majority of these institutions were privately owned and funded, and "many of the individual creators of black hospitals and nurse training schools acted out of a complex array of motives ... altruism, professional self-aggrandizement, or a commitment to the preservation of racial segregation" (Hine, 1989, pp. 9–10).

As White female nurses were gaining strides related to education, autonomy, and work conditions, the image and role of the Black nurse was still associated with servitude and obligation. Students and graduate nurses "constituted an indispensable, loyal, and unpaid labor force" (Hine, 1989, p. 35). White nurse educators and administrators were concerned that Black nurses could not meet the rigors of education and that they would not have the ability to manage the knowledge or skills they would be taught. Black nurses still suffered from stereotypes associated with their racial origins. The quality of Black students' work and their commitment to the profession were questioned, as well as their ability to be trained. "It has [been] demonstrated ... that while backward or underprivileged people may want ... help, they do not always welcome guidance and direction" (Hine, 1989, p. 33). This senti-ment continued for years as opportunities for Black nursing students were limited; they were often the first to be fired and the last to be hired during the Depression and into World War II (Hine, 1989).

Concern over poorly prepared students initiated a debate that contin-ues today related to what is the best education type and what qualifications should determine entry into practice. Attempts to standardize education resulted in diploma programs administered through hospital schools and degree programs provided by colleges and universities. As educational pro-grams were expanded many options for degrees became available. With concerns over shortages of nurses after the war, nursing aid programs still flourished as well.

Graduate nurses and student nurses encountered difficulties coexist-ing in the hospital setting since the majority of patients preferred student nurses over the staff nurse. It was determined that student nurses provided the majority of the nursing care, and staff nurses were only a small per-centage of the hospital's employees. "Was a good system one that allowed exploitation of student nurses to subsidize the cost of patient care or was it a system designed to maximize preparation of quality nurses?" (Kalisch & Kalisch, 2004, p. 240). Through efforts to improve education, graduate nurses regained a position of importance, and relationships between stu-dent nurses and staff nurses improved some.

Licensure and Regulation

THE LICENSURE AND REGULATION ASPECT of nursing throughout the 1920s to the 1940s was one of turmoil as the nation dealt with many social issues at the beginning of the 1920s and then attempted to recover through the 1930s from the great financial collapse in 1929. From the early 1900s into the early 1920s, great effort was made to promote licensure and regulating bodies for nurses in all states. Regulation became an issue as the various schools differed in their curriculums and the quality of nurses com-pleting their programs:

> Nursing's biggest problems were to bring some order to the chaos of unregu-
> lated and widely differentiated schools, of reducing the overproduction of

poorly prepared nurses, and of providing supplemental educational offerings to nurses who had been trained in substandard programs ... the public must face this situation and see that the same kind of pubic support given to normal schools and agricultural colleges [is needed] ... it has cost the public practically nothing to produce nurses ... nurses [even pay] for their own education ... without some kind of radical treatment, it is doubtful if the nursing body can get back into a healthy condition. (Stewart, 1931, pp. 609–610)

Sophia Palmer worked for 20 years to help nurses understand the need for state registrations:

We frequently hear from or talk with nurses who we realize have failed to grasp ... the reasons for this movement ... to comprehend something of how such registration will affect the nurse already in practice ... it is the first great concerted effort of nurses for the advancement, elevation, and protection of the nurses of the future ... with all the advance, the trained nurse of today has no legal standing or right to call herself a trained nurse before the law ... a strong concerted action is needed to improve the educational standard, to protect the public and nurses themselves against impostors, and to give trained nurses a place among the honorable professions! (Donahue, 1996, p. 331)

The efforts related to licensure and regulation during that period of time were, in reality, attempts to regulate education such that state boards of nursing could rely on universal standards of preparation as the student obtained either a diploma certificate or a graduation certificate from an acceptable training program. There were continued endeavors to regulate licensure through standard examinations that were mandatory in order for a license to be issued. As licensing for nurses became a reality in 48 states, nurse representation on boards was authorized through legislation, allowing for nurses to judge the competency of other nurses. From state to state, regulations varied concerning the title of registered nurse; requirements were not mandatory, and some "denied untrained individuals the use of the registered nurse (RN) title; others specified a time period when qualified trained nurses were eligible for registration without examination" (Donahue, 1996, p. 331). Early nurse regulations supported nurse practice acts, which defined nursing roles and responsibility, created uniformity in nursing schools, strengthened collaboration among nurses, furthered nurse organizations, and supported, nurse licensure laws (Donahue, 1996).

Nursing examinations were written by the individual states during the 1930s. Many of the tests were not effective tools in measuring knowledge or preparation of those who took them. As more nurses were trained and prepared for the profession of nursing, it became apparent that nurses should be licensed soon after completing their educational program and that a national test would be more effective in determining adequate preparation. In the early 1940s, the National League for Nursing proposed a test bank of questions taken from individual state board-submitted questions to develop a national test for nurses.

Nursing Research

SIGMA THETA TAU WAS FOUNDED in Indianapolis in the early 1920s when six nursing students felt that scholarship and research would promote the profession of nursing and bring greater recognition. This organization became an honor society for nursing, and membership was based on scholarly ability and leadership. The nurses who started this organization chose the name based on the Greek words for love, honor, and courage. Sigma, Theta, and Tau are the alphabet letters starting each of those words – Storgé, Tharsos, and Timé (STTI, 2008). Baccalaureate and graduate students were and still are eligible candidates along with community nurses and leaders. Over time, the organization became a society for international nurse scholarship and is now known as Sigma Theta Tau International. Nursing research and leadership have advanced as a result of their efforts during the last 80 years.

During the 1930s, the Association of Collegiate Schools of Nursing was formed to advance education and promote research related to educational criteria. Goals were aimed at changing the professional level of the nurse from that of one who is trained to do certain functions to that of one who could use acquired knowledge. "Because of the different types of programs offered by these schools, it was necessary to set up different standards for the schools offering combined academic and basic professional programs" (Stewart, 1936, pp. 45–46). The association's declaration identified how the student's preparation at a hospital nursing school differed from that of an institution of higher learning, "the latter ... preparing graduate nurses for specialized work as teachers, supervisors, or administrators of nursing schools" (Stewart, pp. 45–46). Preparation in an academic setting encouraged the student to view nursing differently and eventually supported examination of the way students were prepared and how that preparation impacted the care they provided. Schools that met curriculum principles fulfilled membership requirements and were eligible to participate in the organization, which eventually became an accrediting agency for nursing institutions. The Association of Collegiate Schools of Nursing pointed out the need for research in nursing, and more specifically, the need to prepare nurse researchers to scrutinize all aspects of the profession from instruction to practice.

Over the next 20 years the organization advanced the profession of nursing as it cultivated interest in nursing research in order to become equal with other departments in the college and university setting. It encouraged the American Nurses Association to publish a magazine with a focus on research; the journal eventually became known as *Nursing Research*. Over time it merged with the National League for Nursing Accrediting Commission, a division of the National League for Nursing, responsible for accreditation of associate degree, diploma, baccalaureate, master's, and licensed practical nursing programs for all the United States and its territories (Donahue, 1996).

Nurses in the community continued to intervene in the lives of their patients as they advocated for better health while documenting improved outcomes. Although their research from the 1920s to the 1940s was perhaps somewhat informal, they shared interventions related to education, treatments, patient care, specific diseases, and populations of interest such as women and children. They described specific results from those interventions and made recommendations regarding care based on those observations. During the following era, research became more formalized and nurse researchers and theorists emerged to the benefit of the profession.

Summary

THE YEARS FROM 1920 TO 1940 were not as eventful as the first 20 years of the century with regard to changes in nursing. The country had ended one war and the next had not yet started, so there was little progress related to nursing and the military. Efforts of nurse leaders slowed as women gained rights and the economy boomed and then crashed. Scientific endeavors continued and innovation focused on radios, small appliances, telephone systems, mechanical automation, air transportation, and other similar technologies. Medical advances were focused on epidemiology, vaccination, and the use of antibiotics to control infections.

The majority of progress during this time for nurses was linked to educational standards and the promotion of nursing organizations that could and did advance nursing as a profession. The role of the nurse changed through acquisition of cognitive aptitude associated with technical skill proficiency. The nursing process had not yet been described, but many were using the various aspects of that concept to determine nursing issues and to suggest solutions and actions that improved nursing then and continued to do so.

⦿ IDEAS FOR FURTHER EXPLORATION

1. What effect did the Great Depression have on nurses in general? How did it change the ability of nurses to do that which they had been prepared to do?

2. Learn more about Black nurses who served their community as effectively as they could. What were their facilities like (schools and hospitals)? How did their training compare or contrast to that of peer nurses who were not Black. What organizations, if any, promoted their cause, and how did they do this?

3. During the 1920s to the 1940s, there were many ideas about nurse training and education. Research historical records to learn about some of those issues and ideas not mentioned in this text. Consider how these recommendations or changes impacted nursing practice during the next several decades.

✦ DISCUSSION QUESTIONS: APPLICATION TO CURRENT PRACTICE

1. What organizations affected the future of nursing then and now? What were the implications? Did they advance the profession of nursing? Why or why not?

2. What did women's suffrage do for nurses? Did feminist ideas really help nurses? Why or why not? How did this impact the socialization of male nurses then and now?

3. Hospital nurses became more prevalent during this time, yet the majority of nurses still provided care in the community. Explore what community nurses did then and what they do now. Describe some benefits to the community from these nurses then and now.

✦ MeSH SEARCH TERMS

Education, nursing
Home nursing
Public health nursing
World War II

Other useful non-MeSH terms:

Frontier nursing
National Council for War Service
Sigma Theta Tau

Association of Collegiate Schools of
　　Nursing
National League for Nursing

⧊ SUGGESTED READING

Abel, E. K. (2000). *Hearts of wisdom: American women caring for kin, 1850–1940.* Cambridge, MA: Harvard University Press.

Brainard, A. M. (1985). *The evolution of public health nursing.* New York: Garland.

Breckinridge, M. (1952). *Wide neighborhoods: A story of the Frontier Nursing Service.* New York: Harper.

Brinkley, A. (2003). *American history: A survey* (11th ed.). New York: McGraw-Hill.

Buhler-Wilkinson, K. (2001). *No place like home: A history of nursing and home care in the United States.* Baltimore: Johns Hopkins University Press.

Ettinger, L. E. (2006). *Nurse-midwifery: The birth of a new American profession.* Columbus: Ohio State University Press.

⧊ REFERENCES

Allen, S. K., & Semba, R. D. (2002). The trachoma "menace" in the United States, 1897–1960. *Survey of Ophthalmology, 47*(5), 500–509.

Andrist, L. C., Nicholas, P. K., & Wolf, K. A. (Eds.). (2006). *A history of nursing ideas.* Sudbury, MA: Jones and Bartlett.

Brinkley, A. (2003). *American history: A survey* (11th ed.). New York: McGraw-Hill.

Donahue, M. P. (1996). *Nursing: The finest art* (2nd ed.). St. Louis, MO: Mosby.

Dublin, L. L. (1932). *The first one thousand midwifery cases of the Frontier Nursing Service.* New York: Metropolitan Life Insurance Company.

Faria, M. A. (2002). Medical history—hygiene and sanitation. *Medical Sentinel, 7*(4), 122–123.

Goodnow, M. (1943). *Nursing history in brief.* (2nd ed. rev.). Philadelphia: W.B. Saunders.

Hall, C. M. (1929). Effect of the grading committee report on schools of nursing. *American Journal of Nursing, 29*(2), 129–134.

Hine, D. C. (1989). *Black women in white: Racial conflict and cooperation in the nursing profession, 1890–1950.* Bloomington: Indiana University Press.

Houweling, L. (2004). Image, function, and style: A history of the nursing uniform. *American Journal of Nursing, 104*(4), 40–48.

Kalisch, P. A., & Kalisch, B. J. (2004). *American nursing: A history* (4th ed.). Philadelphia: Lippincott, Williams, and Wilkins.

Mosby, Inc. (2000). *Nursing reflections: A century of caring.* St. Louis, MO: Mosby.

O'Lynn, C. E., & Tranbarger, R. E. (Eds.). (2007). *Men in nursing: History, challenges, and opportunities.* New York: Springer.

Sanger, M. (1922). *The pivot of civilization.* New York: Brentano's.

Sigma Theta Tau International (STTI). (2008). *Organizational Fact Sheet.* Accessed July 23, 2008, from http://www.nursingsociety.org/aboutus/mission/Pages/factsheet.aspx

Stewart, I. M. (1931). Trends in nursing education. *American Journal of Nursing, 31*(5), 601–611.

Stewart, I. M. (1936). The Association of Collegiate Schools of Nursing. *American Journal of Nursing, 36*(1), 45–47.

CHAPTER 7

Nursing in the United States From the 1940s to the Early 1960s

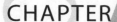

1943
- Nurse Training Act passed, making free training for nurses available
- Streptomycin introduced as the first remedy for tuberculosis
- Use of the Pap smear established
- First class of Army Nurse Corps flight nurses graduate

1945
- First Mobile Army Surgical Hospital (MASH) units established
- Penicillin produced for medical use

1949
- American Birth Control League created
- Association of Colored Graduate Nurses becomes part of the American Nurses Association (ANA)

1940	1941	1942	1943	1944	1945	1946	1947	1948	1949

1940
First blood bank established

1942
- Federal training funds for nurses ($3 million) approved
- Nurses held as prisoners of war by the Japanese during World War II (Angels of Bataan)

1946
- Communicable Disease Center established (later, Centers for Disease Control and Prevention)
- Dr. Benjamin Spock publishes *Baby and Child Care*

1948
World Health Organization established

1939–1945 World War II

1940s • Advent of mass-produced antibiotics

PROFESSIONALISM, EDUCATIONAL REFORMATION, AND ACCEPTANCE OF MINORITY NURSES

Deborah M. Judd

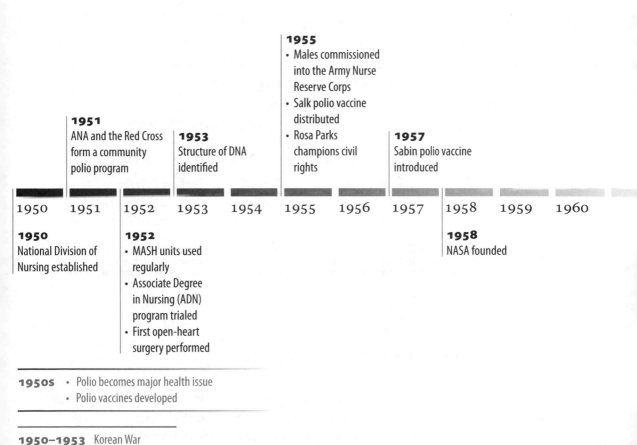

1955
- Males commissioned into the Army Nurse Reserve Corps
- Salk polio vaccine distributed
- Rosa Parks champions civil rights

1951
ANA and the Red Cross form a community polio program

1953
Structure of DNA identified

1957
Sabin polio vaccine introduced

| 1950 | 1951 | 1952 | 1953 | 1954 | 1955 | 1956 | 1957 | 1958 | 1959 | 1960 |

1950
National Division of Nursing established

1952
- MASH units used regularly
- Associate Degree in Nursing (ADN) program trialed
- First open-heart surgery performed

1958
NASA founded

1950s
- Polio becomes major health issue
- Polio vaccines developed

1950–1953 Korean War

OUR NURSING HERITAGE: KEY PEOPLE

Frances P. Bolton	Was not a nurse, but was a wealthy Congresswoman and a nursing supporter
	Proposed the first national house bill for nurse training
Luther Christman	Encouraged science-based education
	Promoted use of best clinical practices
	Founded the American Association for Men in Nursing
Ruth L. Johnson (and her peer consultants)	Consultant for U.S. Public Health Services
	Managed and monitored nurse education funded by government
Lucile Petry Leone	Served as the first Assistant Surgeon General
	Founding director of the Cadet Nurse Corps
Hildegard Peplau	Early nurse researcher
	Pioneer of psychiatric and mental health nursing
	Wrote *Interpersonal Relations in Nursing*, in which she introduced the concept of the nurse–patient relationship
Dorothy Reilly	Wrote the *Quick Nurse Reference Book for Nurses*
	Encouraged educational standards during World War II
	Recipient of many National Institutes of Health grants for educational innovations

Note: Many of the nurses listed in the previous chapter(s) continued to influence nursing during this era.

Sociopolitical Climate

WORLD WAR II HAD GREAT impact on the United States, whose relationships with countries across both oceans changed dramatically. Following the surprise Japanese attack on Pearl Harbor, major changes occurred in the lives of all Americans. Never before in that century had Americans felt so threatened and astonished as life changed in a matter of a few minutes, such that it would never be the same. Over the next several years there were numerous important changes in daily living, technology, economics, sociopolitical realms, global relationships, science, and more importantly for this review, nursing and medical practices. As Americans were beginning to recover from the Great Depression, the demands of war provided a tremendous stimulus for the economy with the creation of numerous jobs and opportunities.

When Hitler invaded Poland and Czechoslovakia in 1939, Japan had already invaded China, and most of the Baltic states had likewise been overrun by the Soviet Union. President Franklin Roosevelt tried to maintain neutrality during these crises, avoiding commitments that required financial and political support outside of the United States. He supported actions and programs of the League of Nations—which had been created earlier to deal with global issues—while avoiding obligations outside U.S. borders as his predecessors had. Since a recession created financial concerns, the administration focused its efforts on developing domestic programs that improved conditions for those who were still suffering the effects of the Depression. U.S. policies changed when totalitarian governments came too close to home (Brinkley, 2003).

Roosevelt had just conceived the New Deal, which created many of the social and welfare programs we still know in hopes that the country's confidence in general would be restored and that life in America might become better. These programs were issued in an era during which government became involved in the regulation of economic measures and had great influence on political ideas and programs. Although the New Deal was only partially successful in eliminating poverty, changing unemployment, improving the economy, and changing people's lives, most Americans believed that government should continue be involved in protecting the economy and providing protection for all (Brinkley, 2003).

The attack on Hawaii necessitated new strategy and foreign policy along with war preparation. The battleship *Arizona* was hit numerous times and sank along with four other ships into the bay at Pearl Harbor. Casualties associated with this attack numbered about 2,400. There were about 82 military nurses stationed at the three military facilities near Pearl Harbor. Civilian and military nurses served diligently and delivered superb care to all who required it; over the course of the war more than 60,000 nurses provided nursing care to their patients. Sixty-seven army nurses and 11 navy nurses in the Philippines were captured during the Japanese invasion and kept as prisoners of war; they became known as the Angels of Bataan. Some navy nurses were also captured in Guam and held as prisoners of war (Wilson, 1996).

During the war, women played a major role in preparing and supporting the nation. Women left their homes and families to work in a variety of occupations. By the end of the war, about one third of all women worked outside the home. Each of the respective military corps recruited women during the war to serve in their reserves corps for women; the jobs they filled were those vacated by men, who were sent abroad or recruited into military service. The hundreds of thousands of women who worked in these noncombat occupations were sometimes referred to as Rosie the Riveter, since many of them worked in plants and factories. As women participated specifically in military roles, some worried that they were not suited for this type of life; however, by the end of the war, the country knew that it could not have accomplished what it did without this female dedication.

The Image of Nursing

NURSES WERE RESPECTED, REVERED AND considered professionals; they were portrayed in recruitment posters with slogans such as these from the National Archives and Records Administration World War II Nursing Recruitment posters:

- "Be a Cadet Nurse: the girl with a future; A Lifetime Education FREE" (Donahue, 1996, p. 372)

- "YOU ARE NEEDED NOW: join the ARMY NURSE CORPS" (U.S. Army Nurse Corps, 1943)

- "Enlist in a proud profession!: Join the U.S. Cadet Nurse Corps" (U.S. Public Health Service, 1943)

- "From now on it's YOUR job: There is a place for EVERY woman in this nurse crisis"
  (National Archives and Records Administration, n.d.)

During periods of war, nurses had always been present; however, it wasn't until World War II that they attained a positive national status.

Serving in embattled lands whose names the public has never heard before, in hospital ships on all the seas, and in air ambulances evacuating the wounded by plane, the nurse came into her own as comforter and healer. Femininity in foxholes, with mud-caked coveralls over pink panties, captured the imagination of the public and the fighting men of America. (Robinson, 1946, p.358)

More than 50,000 army nurses served on or near the battlefields, and they are remembered for their contributions and bravery. When serving on the front they wore coveralls or fatigues; in the field they often wore shirt-dresses with sturdy shoes for comfort and utility. Of course, female military nurses wore the uniform of their respective service, which was similar to the male servicemen's uniform. As was the style for women of the day, a skirt or dress, rather than pants, was required. Wearing of their formal attire was limited while serving in a war zone; they wore uniforms that fit their duties, with fatigues or surgical scrubs serving as their utilitarian attire. The following image was reported by a soldier who worked side by side with these female nurses:

They were 24 hours with plenty of things dropping all around—planes being shot down. Let me tell you they quickly learned to dig foxholes. I have seen them digging them with a spoon—two things they soon learn to do—wear helmets and dig foxholes.... They had no water except in their canteens when unloaded. [When I arrived] they welcomed me with food and equipment. They had no tents. Each nurse was given one blanket and half shelter tent, their "B" and "C" rations and a musette bag. They were wearing fatigues and steel helmets. They used the ground for their bed—but they were there ready to go and waiting for us when the situation demanded it. (Aynes, 1973, p. 245)

Student nurses in a hospital or academic program wore black hose, sturdy black shoes, and a dark colored dress with white cuffs, a white collar, and a white apron. After 3 years of schooling they received their white caps, and white bibs became their aprons; these were very rewarding achievement symbols. During their senior year they received the coveted black ribbons or bands to place on their caps. Once school was completed, they could wear the white dress along with white hose and white shoes, which was attire that symbolized nursing (Mosby, Inc., 2000). Student nurses might still be called probies during their first several months of training. They were required to wear a student uniform from early morning to late at night. Some complained of the stiffness of the starched collar to peers, but felt privileged for the educational opportunities and prospect of future employment.

The student military nurses were provided the striking gray street military uniform, which consisted of a suit jacket, a skirt, red shoulder epaulets and a jaunty beret. They were provided a gray wool uniform for winter and two gray and white striped cotton summer uniforms; the novel beret was worn with either uniform. They wore a black belted coat in winter and a gray raincoat in the summer, and had an oval shoulder handbag. Nurses were required to provide their own blouses, shoes, and stockings; shoes were to be durable, and it was recommended that they only purchase one pair since most used ration coupons for their nonissue pieces of the uniform (United States Public Health Service, Division of Nurse Education, 1944). These students did not have to pay for their clinical and academic training if they agreed to serve the nation as nurses either in a military situation or in a civilian hospital during the war .

The Education of Nurses

DURING WORLD WAR II, THE Cadet Nurse Program of the United States contributed much to the curriculum and educational structure of both military and civilian nursing programs of the nation. The Nurse Training Act passed in 1943 provided money for nurse education in any military or civilian school. The appropriated funds allowed for each nursing student to receive free tuition, uniforms, and any school fees required; those who qualified might also obtain a stipend during training. All nursing schools were advised to develop a 36-month basic nurse education program so that they could be trained adequately and in an efficient period of time (Robinson & Perry, 2001). The surgeon general of the United States, along with the National Council for War Nursing, became responsible for coordination and determination of educational program goals anywhere in the United States. Surgeon General Thomas Parran pointed out that the federal curriculum pattern was just a guide:

> ... schools of nursing are free to select students, to plan curricula, and to formulate policies consistent with the Act and the traditions of the institutions

concerned.... I am confident that through continued teamwork we shall achieve the goal, which means so much to the health of our nation. (as cited in Robinson & Perry, 2001, p. 7)

Candidates who joined military nursing schools were obligated to serve during the entire length of World War II; their service could be as a civilian nurse or as a military nurse. Any state accredited school would be eligible for Nurse Training Act funds if it established an accelerated program and required graduate students to finalize their education with a 6-month clinical residency in a civilian or federal hospital. Nurses could also choose to serve as a public health nurse to meet their residency requirement. United States Public Health Service nurses were instrumental in providing nurse educators with workshops designed to provide information on the best ways to teach nursing students. Additionally, they helped hospitals and nursing schools determine a budget for each educational program. These regional nurse representatives became consultants to the directors of the school of nursing, guiding them through curriculum development and educational standards as they implemented programs that would become eligible for the nurse training funds (Robinson & Perry, 2001).

Before a school could be accredited to participate, its curricula, practice hours, lecture hours, and health and guidance clinical plan had to be reviewed.

It was necessary for the federal and state agencies to work together because the state boards of nurse examiners varied widely from state to state, which was a concern ... with the accelerated program of the Corps, graduating nurse cadets had to meet the requirements of their licensing agency [in addition to the funding standard]. We emphasized education of the students. (Robinson & Perry, 2001, pp. 14–15)

In order to facilitate coordination and cooperation of the nurse directors, nurse consultants emphasized the benefits of such a program during the war but more importantly the community benefits after the war (Robinson & Perry, 2001).

Becoming a nurse still required an unselfish commitment to serving fellow beings; a certain degree of sacrifice during the educational process, clinical residency, and future nurse service was required. Students in hospital nursing schools not only participated in nursing education, but were frequently required to work as housekeepers or orderlies since there were not enough personnel to fill those positions. These hospital-based probationers were required to take introduction to nursing and the practice of nursing procedures; if they did not pass these courses with appropriate grades, they were dismissed from the program and others were recruited to take their place. Their peers in the college or university setting took similar courses during their first quarter of school and likewise had to receive a passing grade in order to continue in their program. Stringent requirements were set in order to utilize educational funds as best possible. "We carried 20 credit hours of coursework the first 3 months and had to maintain a C average ..." (Robinson & Perry, 2001, p. 69). Once they completed the introductory term, they became precadets.

> Pre-cadets worked split shifts; 7 to 10 a.m., off to class at the university, back to the hospital for duty 7–10 pm..., then to the dorm to study. Many nights we studied until 2 am.... We had to learn so many facts ... (Robinson & Perry, 2001, p. 69)

Nurse candidates who participated in a program that was associated with the Nurse Funding Act were enlisted into military service and required to take the nurse cadet pledge, which reviewed their obligation to follow their instructors and their physician peers faithfully, to keep themselves healthy and alert, and to remember their promise to serve their country as a nurse during the entire war. Once they began their schooling, they were required to acquire certain military skills:

> Although not a military organization, knowledge of military carriage and the significance of wearing a uniform with pride and distinction will be a valuable asset to its members. By improving posture, so important to a nurse who must be on her feet many hours of the day, the military drill should help cadet nurses in their work. (Robinson & Perry, 2001, p. 55)

Several cadet nurses captured their experiences with military training in the following excerpts:

> I joined 100 cadet nurses at St. Paul Methodist Church.... When asked to stand at attention, the rustle of our starched aprons brought smiles to attending guests. We wore our hospital uniforms with the Maltese patch on our shoulders.... We didn't know the first thing about marching.... Drill sergeants

were called out from local military bases to teach the cadet nurses to march correctly.... Pick up a rock and carry it in your right hand ... but we still had a hard time telling our right foot from the left! ... The language ... and the impatience of the sergeants scared us, however we turned out to be a striking addition to military parades.... The official flag of the U.S. Nurse Corps featured the symbol of the Maltese cross. We looked to [it] as a symbol of united strength, loyalty, honor, and heroic sacrifice ... I had a deep feeling of thankfulness and pride in my chosen profession. On stage 48 cadet nurses stood before the flags of the different states [and] a cadet nurse guarded our impressive flag with the caduceus ... another stood watch over the new banner of the Corps with the silver Maltese cross blazing in a center of red. (Robinson & Perry, 2001, pp. 55–65)

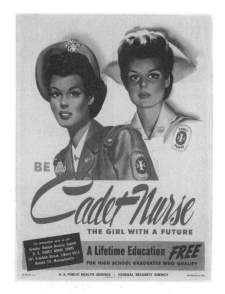

"Be a Cadet Nurse: The girl with a future; A Lifetime Education FREE for high school graduates who qualify" Poster by Jon Whitcomb

Advances in Nursing Practice

I T WAS IN THE EARLY 1940s when the use of antibiotics began to alter the outcomes of common diseases such as pneumonia, syphilis, tuberculosis, whooping cough, and gastric infections. Louis Pasteur, Alexander Fleming, Robert Koch, and others described the phenomena of germs and the idea that some organisms could be used favorably to eliminate disease rather than promote it. As penicillin use became more frequent there were significant decreases in mortality rates, especially associated with pneumonia. Antibiotics, of course, were not without undesirable effects, but generally the benefits far outweighed the disadvantages. Sensitivity to penicillin was initially one of the most concerning issues of its widespread use; however, in future decades, new variations and classes of antibiotics helped to alleviate this concern (Kalisch & Kalisch, 2004).

When Florey and Chain developed an antibiotic form of penicillin, it revolutionized medical care; it offered medical providers something to use for best wound management, surgery, respiratory infections, and other infectious diseases. It was valuable during the war as countless soldiers survived wounds they would not have survived during previous wars. In the 1940s, it was mass produced, permitting more than 7 million individuals to receive it for a variety of medical conditions. Also at this time, Charles Drew, an African American physician, perfected the technique of blood donations for transfusion and opened the first blood bank in the United States in 1940. Despite his role in this endeavor, he personally could not donate, nor could other African Americans, due to continued issues with segregation. Three years later, Selman Waksman introduced streptomycin, the first antibiotic found to be successful in the treatment of tuberculosis, which was still a very common disease in the United States. Tuberculosis, which had been the third-leading cause of death in the 1920s, became less problematic, and by the mid 1940s it had fallen to be the seventh-leading cause of death nationally (Kalisch & Kalisch, 2004). In 1943, the Papanicolaou (Pap) smear was introduced as a means to detect cervical cancer and eventually became a routine test for all women of childbearing age. It was anticipated that this screening mechanism would eventually eliminate cervical cancer, the leading cause of death in women prior to 1940. One year later the first heart surgery for tetralogy of Fallot (blue baby syndrome) was performed when surgeons anastamosed the subclavian and pulmonary arteries, correcting the blood shunt and resultant ischemia (Donahue 1996; Mosby, Inc., 2000).

As the 1950s progressed, care was primarily provided in the hospital setting with most hospitals providing generalized care rather than specialty care. According to Kalisch & Kalisch (2004), the American Medical Association documented that during 1952 over 19 million patients were cared for in the hospital, while 5,600 hospitals provided general medical care and another 1,000 hospitals offered special care for mental health issues or tuberculosis as extended care. The hospitals that conferred specialty care to these long-term patients were primarily supported by tax dollars, since their families frequently did not have financial resources to support the ongoing care required (pp 378–379).

Mosby, Inc. (2000) notes the following reflections about medical and nursing progression during World War II and in the decade that followed (p. 47):

- The National Nursing Council for War Service was founded and became an organization, coordinating war nursing efforts while maintaining nursing endeavors on the home front.

- Military mobile army surgical hospital (MASH) units were created, utilizing both nurses and doctors in a collaborative manner close to the front in order to provide immediate best care possible from injury to surgical or other interventions. They were not readily used during World War II, but they became an essential aspect of medical care for soldiers during the Korean conflict.

- The School of Air Evacuation graduated its first class of flight nurses for the Army Nurse Corps, while a limited number of civilian female pilots participated in military flight endeavors.

- The Communicable Disease Center, later termed the Centers for Disease Control (CDC), was commissioned and operations began in Atlanta, Georgia. This center ultimately participated regularly in medical research, becoming an organization that determines best interventions when new diseases and medical phenomena emerge.

- The United States was introduced to better child rearing techniques when Benjamin Spock's book, *The Common Sense Book of Baby and Child Care*, was released. The book introduced new concepts and was used by many generations of parents.

- The World Health Organization was formed to address global health issues while setting standards and designing worldwide programs to promote healthy living.

As medical technology and innovation continued, many amazing things that had never been done before became ordinary and routine. In 1952, the first open-heart surgery was achieved. The year before this surgery, John Gibbon, Jr. introduced a functioning heart-lung machine—a device that paved the way for this successful cardiac surgery. Surgical accomplishments ensued as did subsequent technological developments to support new procedures; this promoted focused expertise, which ultimately led to specialty care and the design of specialized units within the hospital where care was based on a specific body system, associated organs, and interrelated diseases. By 1960, the artificial kidney was introduced for those who had organ failure, providing a possibility of prolonged life. Other mechanical devices for a variety of diseases and resultant organ failure, including eventual organ replacement, soon followed as novel specialty care techniques were perfected (Donahue 1996; Mosby, Inc., 2000).

As infections that had plagued the United States became generally managed with sulfa, streptomycin, and penicillin antibiotics, acquisition of advanced knowledge concerning disease contagion allowed medical providers of the nation to better manage illness. For example, malaria, which had been very problematic in the South, was finally eradicated through "ditching, draining, dusting, and oiling the breeding waters" of mosquitoes, which carried the malaria (Kalisch & Kalisch, 2004, p. 310). Visiting nurses supervised community health as they monitored and assisted with water supply, milk production, and food supplies in order to promote best health practices and decrease contamination and resultant infections. Programs such as those of the frontier nurse, the rural nurse, or the community nurse promoted educational courses for patients and the community to alleviate the diseases of childhood and childbearing women. In a relatively short period of time, education and access to appropriate care decreased suffering and mortality significantly, while issues associated with aging and disease chronicity became more problematic for society.

Polio became a major health issue by 1950; more than 50,000 Americans were diagnosed with it, and in many communities there were epidemics since the spread of the disease could not be controlled. Nurses in communities banded together with the Red Cross and the National Foundation of Infantile Paralysis to provide care for

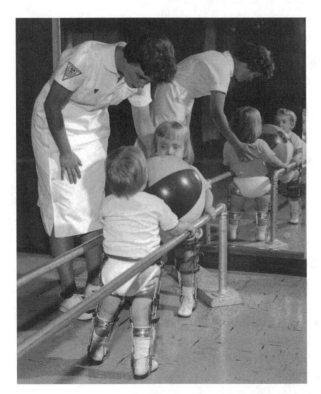

Physical therapist assisting polio-stricken children

those affected and to educate communities on the disease (Donahue 1996; Mosby, Inc., 2000). Significant strides were made during this decade to help eradicate the disease in the United States and even worldwide. Jonas Salk released a killed polio virus vaccine and Albert Sabin later introduced the live oral polio vaccine series. Both of these vaccines were used and the nation initiated mass vaccine administration during the late 1950s. Infants and toddlers were offered immunization, and eventually schoolchildren were required to be vaccinated through community health programs before they could enter neighborhood schools.

Other notable advancements affecting nurses during this decade were (1) the Apgar scoring method, which is still in use today in delivery rooms for assessment of the neonate; (2) the linkage of tobacco use to cancer and other chronic diseases; (3) the identification of the structure of the DNA helix, which enhanced the science of cellular biology and future under-standing of disease at the molecular level; and (4) the discovery of cortisone by Philip Hetch, improving disease management, outcomes, and morbidity levels (Donahue, 1996).

War and Its Effects on Nursing

AFTER THE ATTACK ON PEARL HARBOR in 1941, United States military nurses became a valuable resource in the war efforts once again. Congress, in anticipation of involvement in the war, authorized a million dollars for military nurse training prior to the Pearl Harbor incident; in light of the change in circumstances once the attack occurred, Congress funded another 3 million dollars for nursing education. Kalisch & Kalisch (2004) report the following from the February 1940 *Journal of Nursing*: "Congress, as this is written, had been in session only ten days. The very air is supercharged with tragedy. The war of other countries are profoundly influencing life in our own, and Congress is concerned with ... armaments for defense" (p. 298).

Prior to involvement of the United States in World War II, The National Nursing Council for War was formed, and the rules, regulations, and cur-riculum requirements for war nurses were determined by this organization. During that same period of time, the American Nurses Association, the

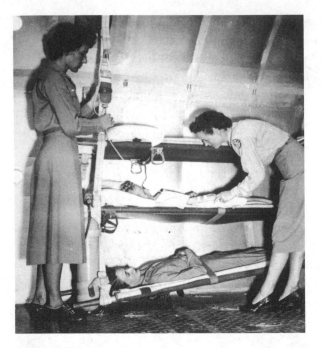

World War II Air Force
Flight Nurses

National League for Nursing Education, and the Army School of Nursing collaborated to support this new
nursing council and the availability of
nurses from all educational institutions in anticipation of nurses being
needed in the near future for military endeavors. Meanwhile, President
Roosevelt initiated the Selective Training and Service Act in 1940, which
required all males aged 21–30 years to
register for the draft. By 1948, all men
aged 18 to 45 years were required to
register; they were eligible for military
service regardless of circumstances.
Emergency funds were mandated for
supplemental public health nurses in
national defense industries, and soon
additional funding was provided for
agencies that could provide commu-
nity defense service to promote health projects in hospitals, schools, and
clinics (Kalisch & Kalisch, 2004; Mosby, Inc., 2000). Prior to the outbreak
of the war there were only about 1,000 nurses in the military corps. The
instantaneous need for nurses was relieved in part by the nursing war council, which encouraged women to consider nursing for the free education and
opportunity (World War II Army Nurse Corps, n.d.).

Nurses during World War II had more options than they did during
World War I. The National Nursing Council on War created two catego-
ries of nursing—that of an armed forces nurse and that of a home service
nurse. War nurse qualifications were defined as a single female below age 40
and not an essential nurse in any organization, including a necessary private
duty assignment. If a nurse met these criteria, then it was suggested she
volunteer for the military nurse corps. If she was married or was needed
to maintain a stateside nursing operation, she would continue service in
the United States, knowing that she was serving her country as best she
could. Nurses took great pride in being able to care for the nation's health

in any capacity that they could. Many nurses eventually joined the ranks of the Army or Navy Nurse Corps.
This caused a severe shortage of nurses in all areas of
nursing and eventually led to some drastic solutions.

Measures were initiated to alleviate the shortage.
Grant funds were approved and marked specifically
for nursing education at state accredited schools and
universities. These funds allowed for nurse refresher
courses, specialty nursing programs, supplementary training, and the new nurse's aide defense training courses. Additionally, minority nurses were
recognized, and the recruitment of Black nurses was
encouraged as the military commissioned the Coordinating Committee on Negro Nursing to campaign
for racial equality in nursing (Donahue, 1996). With
the inclusion of male nurses rather than orderlies into
military nurse corps, another minority group gained
equal opportunities. The inclusion of males and other

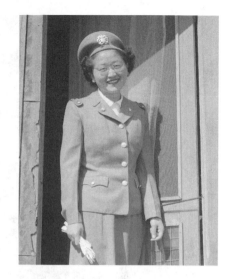

Japanese-American U.S.
Naval Cadet Nurse Kay
Fukuda, by Ansel Adams,
Manzanar Series

minority nurses during this war ultimately affected nursing into the current century as more and more of them were socialized into the profession.
Many male nurses gravitated into specialty areas during World War II and
later wars, and upon return to civilian service, they participated in specialty unit advancement.

Nursing service and responsibilities changed dramatically during World
War II as nurses served on many fronts. They provided service on land,
on sea, and in the air. Their battlefields included over 50 countries, including Africa, Italy, France, Britain, and the islands of the Pacific Rim. As part
of the strategy for military health care, the first MASH was designed, and
MASH units were eventually used widely during combat. Wounded men
were stabilized in the battlefield and then transported to the MASH units
for surgery and other medical interventions. Soldiers were cared for almost
immediately, and this promoted better recovery and reduced mortality.
Nurses served much closer to the front lines and became involved in caring
for patients in a number of different venues, such as Quonset hut clinics
and hospitals, MASH tent hospitals, aboard military ships upon the seas, in
the air as flight nurses, in abandoned buildings at the front, along the trail

World War II military
field hospital

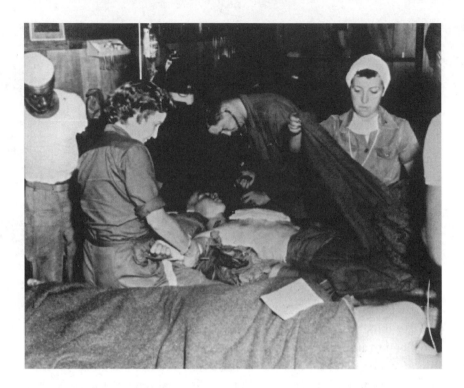

of forced marches, in prison camps, and in a variety of other settings. They proved to be a valuable resource even in very difficult situations.

Nursing care during the war was dependent on nurses who would work until they could work no more; they had a job to do and they did it well. "The sulfonamides, the advent of penicillin, DDT, new developments in anti-malarial therapy, and the ready availability of blood and blood products ... heroism and ingenuity" (Roberts, 1954, p. 344) allowed for nurses and others who cared for patients to obtain favorable outcomes in the face of great obstacles.

As recorded in *The Army Nurse Corps* (Bellafaire, n.d.), men and women from all walks of life experienced a variety of wartime conditions. In the Pacific:

> Eighty-two Army nurses were stationed in Hawaii that infamous morning ... blood-spattered stairs led to hallways where wounded men lay on the floor awaiting surgery. Army and Navy nurses and medics (men trained as orderlies) worked side by side ... a steady stream of seriously wounded

continued to arrive ... [there were] appalling shortages of medical supplies [since they were kept] under lock and key.... Working under tremendous pressure, medical personnel faced shortages of instruments, suture material, and sterile supplies. Doctors performing major surgery passed scissors back and forth from one table to another. Doctors and nurses used cleaning rags as face masks and operated without gloves. (Bellafaire, n.d., pp. 3–4)

In the Philippines:

With each passing week the number of patients in both hospitals increased, and available supplies decreased. Lack of adequate food and clothing left American and Filipino troops susceptible to malaria, dysentery, beriberi, and dengue fever. Increasing numbers of troops suffered from malnutrition ... in each hospital, built to accommodate 1,000 patients, [nurses treated] over 5,000. (Bellafaire, n.d., p. 5)

In Africa:

Each boat carried 5 [Black] nurses, 3 medical officers, and 20 enlisted men. The nurses wore helmets and carried full packs containing musette bags, gas masks, and canteen belts. Only their Red Cross arm bands and lack of weapons distinguished them from fighting troops. They waded ashore ... and huddled behind a sand dune while enemy snipers took potshots.... That evening they found shelter in some abandoned beach houses.... Before the night was over, however, their commanding officer ordered them to an abandoned civilian hospital, where they began caring for invasion casualties. There was no electricity or running water, and the only medical supplies available were those the nurses had.... Doctors operated under flashlights held by nurses ... wounded soldiers lay on a concrete floor in pools of blood. Nurses dispensed what comfort they could, although the only sedatives available were the ones that they had carried with them ... [later] nurses sewed over fifty sheets into a large white cross to mark their installation as a hospital to enemy aircraft. (Bellafaire, n.d., pp. 9–10)

In the air:

While in flight the nurse watched for anxiety attacks because many soldiers had never flown before. [She] applied bandages and dressings, relieved pain, administered oxygen, and cared for those who became airsick. A bout of airsickness could be fatal to a patient with a broken jaw that had been wired shut. Nurses often gave patients enough medication to encourage sleep throughout the trip. Some soldiers suffering from "battle fatigue" were so emotionally disturbed that they had to travel under restraint. (Bellafaire, n.d., p.15)

In Italy:

[We] saw increasing numbers of soldiers with malaria. Nurses lined the tents with mosquito netting in an attempt to control the spread of the disease through the hospital, but eventually medical personnel also succumbed. Despite the malaria epidemic, nurses at this hospital worked 12-hour shifts ... [nurses] handled a spectrum of wounds including head, chest, and orthopedic, as well as shock ... the hospital would admit 300 patients in one 24-hour period and evacuate 200 to North Africa for further treatment. Most patients went by train to the coast where they were placed on hospital ships. Critically ill patients were evacuated by plane. (Bellafaire, n.d., p. 16)

In Europe:

Evacuation hospitals followed the troops through France. Transportation facilities were strained to the limit, and the unit encountered frequent delays. They often slept out in the open without tents. Their experience alternated between periods of exhausting activity and intense boredom. They had to be flexible, innovative, quick-thinking, patient, adaptable, and highly skilled ... [nurses cared for prisoners of war] victims of starvation, with long-neglected wounds inflicted by systematic torture, many also suffered from typhus, frozen feet, gangrene, bed sores, and severe dermatitis. Eight out of every ten inmates had tuberculosis. Despite intensive care, many died from weakness, malnutrition, and disease. (Bellafaire, n.d., p. 24)

Nursing Workforce Issues

BY 1940, THERE WERE ONLY four all-male nursing schools in the United States. The Mills Training School for Men opened in 1888, and it eventually became part of the Bellevue Schools of Nursing in 1929 when the female and male nursing schools that were associated with Bellevue Hospital joined together; both schools had diploma programs at that time. The school closed during the 1960s with the demise of many diploma programs. The Alexian Brothers Nursing Schools in Saint Louis and Chicago were associated with a Catholic order of nursing dating back to the 10th century. These schools trained nurses initially for the care of the dying patients or sick men in their community; many of the graduates worked as private duty or psychiatric nurses. The male trainees had to be a member of the congregation and were identified as brothers; after graduation they continued to provide care to the sick and the poor. The Pennsylvania Hospital School of Nursing for Men was founded in 1914, about 30 years after the establishment of the women's school of nursing. When the Pennsylvania schools were established, nursing care in the hospital setting was segregated nationally by gender; female nurses cared for female patients while male nurses who were identified as orderlies cared only for male patients. Pennsylvania Hospital's nursing program was one of the first to allow female nurses to care for male patients; however, it did not allow males to care for females in most circumstances. As nursing education changed during the 1970s, many diploma programs were forced to cease operations, including Pennsylvania Hospital's programs (O'Lynn & Tranbarger, 2007).

Male nursing opportunities and nursing education were still limited; of the 28,000 nurses who graduated in 1940, only 212 men graduated from the four male nursing schools while an additional 710 graduated from coed programs. That was roughly 10 male students from each of the 70 institutions that admitted male students. As the nursing shortage during the war created a need for nurses at home and abroad, men were more attracted to the field of nursing. Kalisch & Kalisch (2004) actually coined the phrase, "the harassed male nurse" when discussing issues of male gender and nursing until the 1950s (p. 373). Craig (1940) suggests that despite acceptance of some males into a few established nursing institutions, in reality there were significant restrictions placed on males, and they were actually discriminated against, not unlike females who attempted to enter the medical field to become physicians. He further recounts:

> [There were] opportunities that awaited well qualified men ... the increased need for nurses to have scientific knowledge and skills and the fact that tasks now unrelated to nursing, were delegated to aides ... the work of the nurse [is] now more interesting and satisfying ... Advisors [should] carefully consider the personality, character, and ability of the prospective student. He needs to be versatile in his interests and to possess a considerable degree of leadership ... Nursing is not a profession for a poorly adjusted or

inadequate person ... The young man who is well liked and respected by his fellows and by older men is the most likely to succeed ... opportunities awaiting men of such caliber are private duty nursing, institutional nursing, industrial nursing, and special [nursing] fields. (pp. 666–667)

Support for male nurses in the military was sponsored by both the American Nurses Association and the American Hospital Association, since licensure and regulations at the state level stipulated standards for practice, registration, and licensure. As a result of inquiry and letters of support, a bill was introduced in 1950 that allowed for commission of males into the military as a nurse; it wasn't until 1955 that the bill was finally passed. Of great concern to these male nurses was their classification as an orderly despite their formal training as a registered nurse; an orderly was paid half as much as the nurses were. Once commissioned, pay increased and was comparable to that of a female nurse in the military ("Proud to Serve," n.d.).

By 1960, only 1% of all registered nurses were male since most nursing schools still did not admit them as students, despite military recognition of their services. Prior to the end of the 1950s, nursing and teaching were considered female professions, and males were not encouraged to enter either one of those fields. Despite the long-standing history of males caring for patients in a multitude of wars over several centuries, the male nurse became a rarity in hospital and community settings.

Nurses who enlisted were concerned about their status in the military related to rank, benefits, pay, and postwar service privileges. In 1942, those who enlisted desired benefits since they were serving their country as were their male peers. "Early in 1941, believing war was imminent, [Sue] volunteered as an Army Nurse. She was at Pearl Harbor when the attack came" (Kalisch & Kalisch, 2004, p. 302). The story about Sue comes from the March, 1944 *Rocky Mountain News*, as quoted in Army Nurse Corps Hearings. Sue eventually became ill and disabled from her war exposures. There were more than 100 other nurses at Fitzsimons Hospital who experienced permanent health changes. Nurses believed that they should be compensated for their losses as were soldiers and others under the same circumstances. Over the next 2 years, continued efforts by the Army Nurse Corps on behalf of these nurses resulted in them receiving temporary officer rank while serving, qualifying for benefits during war service, and entitling them to military benefits for 6 months after the war ended (Kalisch & Kalisch, 2004).

During the entire war there were concerns about the supply of nurses and their ability to manage care in the United States since so many nurses participated in military endeavors. They were eagerly welcomed home. In the meantime, this shortage of nurses led to the formation of nurse's aide training programs throughout the country. These programs were administered through the Office of Civilian Defense and the American Red Cross. Hospitals nationwide were advised to recruit volunteers in order to extend nursing services. The goal was to train 100,000 of them in order to assure that every hospital would have at least one nurse's aide. The intent of the nurse's aide program was to extend the ability of the nurse to perform her duties in any field of service, in the community, or in the hospital. "The deficiency in nursing personnel will be overwhelmingly accentuated if this country becomes involved in defensive combat" ("Training Program," 1941, pp. 44–45) with the anticipated war efforts. The specific criteria developed to guide the preparation of these aides were ("Training Program," 1941):

1. Thorough, specific, and guided intensive training must be completed before one could serve as an aide.

2. Service would be required during the national emergency, and each trained aide would need to serve for a specified number of hours dependent on where he or she was trained to function (clinic, hospital, or community service).

3. Training would be tailored to prepare aides specifically to labor in the organization or nursing discipline in which they would eventually serve.

4. Service was to be provided free of charge; the aides were volunteers who received free training, which was considered their remittance.

5. The aides could not work for the organization they were trained for if they replaced paid nurses; they were only to assist the nurses in their work.

Once the war ended, only one in six nurses returned to their previous nursing positions. This created great concern, and those nurses who had remained in nonmilitary situations could not understand why their peers would not return to hospital, clinic, or community settings. Reasons cited by those who did not wish to return included a desire to marry and start a family, the lack of autonomy in institutions compared to flexible and satisfying roles with great responsibility in the military, and the need for a change due to the intense war experiences. Wages and conditions in hospitals did not seem to meet the professional status that nurses finally believed they had achieved. Many nurses were expected to work like servants for an average of 74 cents per hour, while females in nonnursing jobs were paid more than a dollar an hour. Because of this perceived salary inequity, some nurses became frustrated and dissatisfied.

> You stay on duty until everything is completed, and if you punch the clock an hour or more late, it is apparently your own fault for not being able to plan your work better ... a little more understanding ... kindness, and consideration ... would have prevented the present shortage of nurses ... the daily load carried by each nurse is so heavy that of necessity minor details are neglected so that the important things might be done ... the nurse who is overworked physically, is tense mentally and is made to feel that she is doing nothing ... people expect nurses to be like a high class servant, instead of giving them the status of an actual professional ... (United States Department of Labor, Bureau of Labor Statistics, 1948, pp. 42–43)

Nursing opportunities and responsibilities changed during these decades, eliciting revolutions in healthcare delivery and patient management; these continued far into the future. A focus on better health and more universal access to health care altered education, licensure or credentialing, academic institution accreditation and funding, faculty preparation, and clinical standards, and it promoted nursing research and nursing science. National nursing associations continued to promote the profession while sponsoring standards of practice and defining scope of practice.

Licensure and Regulation

ADVANTAGES OF THE COLLABORATIVE EFFORTS of national nursing organizations were that they transformed standards of education and licensure requirements as they became more universal for all nurses despite the state where they resided or the program in which they were educated. State boards of nursing utilized national standards to help define practice roles and determine qualifications for licensing and standards of regulation. The American Nurses Association, National League for Nursing Education, and the National Organization for Public Health Nursing proposed the following platform to contribute to the development of nursing rules and regulations ("The Biennial," 1946):

1. Improve working and living conditions—minimum salary and a 40-hour workweek.

2. Provide for optimal nursing care for all patients, whether in hospital or community encounters.

3. Allow nurses to participate in implementation and administration of nursing services.

4. Develop nurses' professional organizations for bargaining and negotiation of issues (nonunion).

5. Remove barriers that prevent minority/racial groups from professional development and service.

6. Employ only well-qualified and endorsed nurses or ancillary workers to provide nursing.

7. Facilitate adequate utilization of nurses while providing satisfaction and stability in the workplace.

8. Expand health and medical plans to provide nursing services to the public.

9. Maintain rigid and mandatory educational standards such that nurses participate in initial and continuing education. Allow for educational subsidy to support best practice and outcome.

10. Require periodic evaluation of professional and educational organizations to ensure concerns, issues, and needed actions are addressed.

Nursing Research

THE FEDERAL GOVERNMENT BECAME INVOLVED in promoting the nursing profession through the newly formed Division of Nursing in the early 1950s. This organization later became a division of the Health Resources and Services Administration. It advanced healthcare services for all Americans as more focus was placed on providing quality nursing services. The charge of this government-sponsored administration was to investigate and survey nursing in the United States in order to develop strategies to improve nursing nationally. It looked at how nurses might help provide care to underserved populations; as a result of this endeavor the role of the nurse practitioner and the clinical nurse specialist eventually evolved. Surveys and basic studies were used to determine how nursing was provided, to look at perceived issues and problems, and to correlate conditions with those practices. Several suggestions came forth to help improve nursing practice. Leadership, working conditions, and education were areas where improvements were needed.

The Division of Nursing eventually became the Division of Nursing Resources and was affiliated with the Office of the Surgeon General. It primarily had responsibility for public health nursing and nursing education. There was a cooperative effort to help hospitals and nurses deliver optimum patient care as they looked at staffing and nursing responsibilities in order to avert a nursing shortage and determine if certain activities could be effectively relinquished to others in order to utilize nursing resources most efficiently. Addressing issues of the time, several studies were devised to assess nurse utilization, patient care, patient outcomes, and nurse activity related to nursing and nonnursing functions. Data obtained from studies contributed to meaningful recommendations on how to resolve the challenges that faced the nation related to nursing and the developing shortage in the postwar era.

Hospitals reported nurse shortages by 1950, in part due to women in general (including those already trained as nurses) considering other work options that were perhaps less demanding. An increased number of nurse assistants trained to perform nonessential nursing tasks, accelerated expansion of hospital-based care, and a decline in nursing students after World War II further accentuated the problem. This occurred in a time when scientific endeavors necessitated an increased number of qualified specialty nurses as specialty care expanded. Hospital administrators felt nurses brought on their problems through investigation and explanation: "There is too much talk about 'high professional standards' and not enough about taking care of the sick" (Kalisch & Kalisch, 2004, p. 330). In reality, that was not the case, because nurses worked together through this national nursing shortage (Kalisch & Kalisch, 2004).

The Division of Nursing Resources urged planning for nurse employment and appropriate ways to survey nurses in order to determine a nurse's influence on patient care and health care in general. This information contributed to the notion that nursing research was necessary and important to the development of new ideas and methods. Debate continued over patient acuity, staff ratios, nurse qualifications, and associated resources while the Division of Nursing Resources gathered data to detail the situation. Nursing research was considered by most nursing leaders to be a collaborative effort that was part of the process of quality improvement and problem solving. The identified need for nursing research encouraged female nurses in coming years to describe the science of nursing, the care of nursing, and even the art of nursing.

Summary

MANY ADVANCES IN MEDICAL TECHNOLOGY influenced how nurses cared for patients. The use of antibiotics revolutionized health care and decreased morbidity and mortality. With better ways to care for infections, innovations related to trauma and surgery, and the availability of rapid and effective health care on the front, nurses effected positive outcomes for all. During World War II, they encountered unique medical situations where they utilized their educational background to care for soldiers, civilians, and prisoners remarkably well. They functioned independently, providing that care under difficult circumstances.

Educational advances were the result of government intervention and originality as professional nursing practice was promoted through specific curriculum standards and funding. Nurses nationally were expected to have similar training and licensure, since most nurses were associated with military operations either stateside or abroad. The introduction of nurse's aides alleviated some of the problems associated with the nurse shortage while perhaps changing nursing roles thereafter and creating concerns related to practice standards. Nurses were concerned over continued issues linked to work environment and salary. With acceptance of males and minorities into military nursing corps, segregation in education and practice began to be addressed.

National nursing organizations supported nurses as they recognized and developed a platform that addressed concerns and advances in practice. Rules and regulations were devised so that capability and responsibility were better defined. With the rise of nursing as a profession, the Division of Nursing, a government organization, encouraged research to further the art and science of nursing and caring.

◈ IDEAS FOR FURTHER EXPLORATION

1. Learn more about the military Nurse Corps. How did it influence nursing education and function? Briefly describe two to four aspects of nursing that were affected by them.
2. Assess the implications of routine penicillin and antibiotic use. How did their use revolutionize health care? What effect did they have on morbidity and mortality? List some of these effects.
3. Describe rules and regulations of nursing related to licensure and practice. Were there universal guidelines in the 1940s through the early 1960s? If so, what were they? Compare and contrast them to those of today.

◈ DISCUSSION QUESTIONS: APPLICATION TO CURRENT PRACTICE

1. Learn more about the American nurses' platform of 1946. Along with other national organizations, nurses presented a number of concerns related to nursing. Compile a summary list of three to five of those recommendations. How have these impacted nursing care today? Do these organizations still promote the cause of nurses today? Are the issues the same? If so, which ones?
2. The Division of Nursing was associated with the Health Resources and Service Administration (HRSA) from 1950 until 2000. How did this government agency promote nursing then and now?
3. What advances in biomedical research changed medical or nursing

care? Identify three to five of them. How have they impacted health care since the turn of the 21st century?

✦ MeSH SEARCH TERMS

Antibacterial agents	Mobile health units
Centers for Disease Control and Prevention	Penicillin
Korean War	Poliomyelitis
Military medicine	World Health Organization
Military nursing	World War II

Other useful non-MeSH terms:

"Nurse Training Act"	Cadet nurses
MASH	Division of Nursing

✦ SUGGESTED READING

American Nurses Association. (1994). *50th anniversary, 1944–1994: Enlist in a proud profession! Join the U.S. Cadet Nurse Corps.* Washington, DC: American Nurses Association.

Jackson, K. (2000). *They called them angels: American military nurses of World War II.* Westport, CT: Praeger.

Monahan, E. (2000). *All this hell: U.S. nurses imprisoned by the Japanese.* Lexington: University Press of Kentucky.

Monahan, E., & Neidel-Greenlee, R. (2003). *And if I perish: Frontline U.S. Army nurses in World War II.* New York: Knopf.

Omori, F. (2000). *Quiet heroes: Navy nurses of the Korean War: 1950–1953, Far East command.* Saint Paul, MN: Smith House Press.

Tomblin, B. (1996). *G.I. nightingales: The Army Nurse Corps in World War II.* Lexington: University Press of Kentucky.

❖ REFERENCES

Aynes, E. A. (1973). *From Nightingale to eagle: An army nurse's history.* Englewood Cliffs, NJ: Prentice-Hall, Inc.

Bellafaire, J. A. (n.d.). *The Army Nurse Corps: A commemoration of World War II service.* Retrieved on August 23, 2008, from http://www.history. army.mil/books/wwii/72-14/72-14.htm

The Biennial. (1946). *American Journal of Nursing. 46,* 728–746.

Brinkley, A. (2003). *American history: A survey* (11th ed.). New York: McGraw-Hill.

Craig, L. N. (1940). Opportunities for men nurses. *American Journal of Nursing, 40*(6), 666–670.

Donahue, M. P. (1996). *Nursing: The finest art* (2nd ed.). St. Louis, MO: Mosby.

Kalisch, P. A., & Kalisch, B. J. (2004). *American nursing: A history* (4th ed.). Philadelphia: Lippincott, Williams, and Wilkins.

Mosby, Inc. (2000). *Nursing reflections: A century of caring.* St. Louis, MO: Mosby

National Archives and Records Administration. (n.d.). *From now on it's your job.* Retrieved December 2, 2008, from http://womenshistory.about. com/library/pic/bl_p_wwii_nursing_your_job.htm

O'Lynn, C. E., & Tranbarger, R. E. (Eds.). (2007). *Men in nursing: History, challenges, and opportunities.* New York: Springer.

Proud to serve: The evolution of male Army Nurse Corps officers. (n.d.). Retrieved July 30, 2006 from http://history.amedd.army.mil/ANCWebsite/articles/malenurses.htm

Roberts, M. M. (1954). *American nursing: History and interpretation.* New York: Macmillan.

Robinson, T. M., & Perry, P. M. (2001). *Cadet nurse stories: The call and response of women during World War II.* Indianapolis, IN: Sigma Theta Tau International Honor Society of Nursing, Center Nursing Press.

Robinson, V. (1946). *White caps, the story of nursing.* Philadelphia: Lippincott.

Training program announced for 100,000 nurses' aides. (1941). *Hospital Management, 52,* 44–45.

United States Army Nurse Corps, American National Red Cross. (1943). *You are needed now*. Retrieved December 2, 2008, from http://digital. library.unt.edu/data/rarebooks/posters/001_499/meta-dc-365.tkl

United States Department of Labor, Bureau of Labor Statistics. (1948). *The economic status of registered professional nurses, 1946–1947*. Washington, DC: Government Printing Office.

United States Public Health Service, Division of Nurse Education. (1945, May 7). News release (through Office of War Information) morning newspapers. [RG 90]. Washington, DC: National Archives and Records Administration.

United States Public Health Service, United States Federal Security Agency. (1943). Enlist in a proud profession. Retrieved December 2, 2008, from http://digital.library.unt.edu/data/rarebooks/posters/001_499/meta-dc-606.tkl

Wilson, B. A. (1996). *Women in World War II*. Retrieved August 28, 2008 from http://userpages.aug.com/captbarb/femvets5.html

World War II Army Nurse Corps. (n.d.). Retrieved August 28, 2008, from http://www.u-s-history.com/pages/h1712.html

CHAPTER 8

Nursing in the United States From 1960 to the Early 1980s

1961–1975   Vietnam War

1965–1980   Promotion of advanced practice clinical nurse specialists and nurse practitioners

1961
- Berlin Wall built
- Peace Corps established

1963
President John F. Kennedy assassinated

1969
Man walks on the moon

1960	1961	1962	1963	1964	1965	1966	1967	1968	1969

1962
First research field office for the Department of Nursing opened

1964
- Army Institute of Nursing created at Walter Reed Army Hospital
- Nurse Training Act added to the Public Health Service Act
- Economic Opportunity Act passed to provide poverty assistance
- Cancer linked to smoking for the first time

1966
- American Nurses Association resolution regarding nursing education at institutions of higher education
- Males fully commissioned into Army Nurse Corps

1968
Martin Luther King and Robert Kennedy assassinated

1960–1980 · Specialization of nursing
· Debate over entry level of practice (BSN vs ADN)

DECADES OF CHANGE—REGIONAL CONFLICT, SEGREGATION, AND SPECIALIZATION

Deborah M. Judd

1973
Nursing Diagnoses
National conference

1979
Smallpox considered
eradicated globally
(WHO)

1970	1971	1972	1973	1974	1975	1976	1977	1978	1979	1980

1970
• Computerized axial
  tomography (CAT)
  scanner trialed
• Environmental
  Protection Agency
  (EPA) established

1972
• Watergate
• Equal Rights
  Amendment passed
  by Senate—has yet
  to be ratified

1981
• First HIV
  cases
  identified
• Personal
  computers
  introduced

1982
First Jarvik
artificial heart
implanted

1984
First public
use of the
Internet

1970–1980 Development of advanced computer technology

Early 1980s • NLN publishes a credentialing document and establishes recognized
                   standards for all nursing professionals
                 • First National Council Licensure Exam (NCLEX) given to graduating
                   nurses

1980–1990 Continued innovation in medical research/technology and specialization

1983–1990 Causes of HIV/AIDS identified, treatments defined

OUR NURSING HERITAGE: KEY PEOPLE

Nursing Researchers (not all inclusive)

Virginia Henderson	Defined nursing and nursing concepts
Martha Rogers	Science of Unitary Human Beings
Imogene King	Nursing and patient goal attainment—Theory of Goal Attainment
Ida Orlando	Communications and nursing—Nursing Process Theory
Dorothea Orem	Self-care and self-care deficits
Myra Levine	Conservation and health
Sister Callista Roy	Adaptation and health
Betty Neuman	Expanded consciousness—Systems Model
Margaret Newman	Model of Health
Katherine Kolcaba	Theory of Comfort
Dorothy E. Johnson	Behavioral System Model
Jean Watson	*The Philosophy and Science of Caring*
Maggie Jacobs	Held leadership positions in the largest nurse bargaining unit in the United States in New York City Advocated for the poor and needy (primarily in New York City) Received the Harriet Tubman Award for her community work
Florence S. Wald	Proposed and implemented hospice services in the United States Visiting nurse in New York Visiting Nurse Service Studied death and dying, developed a model for hospice care
Mary Opal Wolanin	Long-term nursing care expert Worked in obstetrics, as well as with Native Americans with tuberculosis Served in the Army Nurse Corps in World War II
Dorothy Smith	Promoted a scientific approach to nursing education Worked for collaboration between nursing service and education Instrumental in promoting advanced nursing practice

Undine Sams	Part of campaign to move the American Nurses Association to Washington, DC, to enable more effective policy-making
	Early supporter of Black nurse membership in state and national nursing organizations
Margretta Madden Styles	Active in global nursing, served as president of the International Council for Nurses
	Defined the role of nursing regulation
	Helped create the American Nurses Credentialing Center (ANCC)

Sociopolitical Climate

THE UNITED STATES WAS GREATLY influenced by global issues during the decades of 1960 and 1970. As the Korean Conflict ended in 1959, relationships with other countries created a number of concerns for the United States government. A Cuban civil revolution occurred shortly after Fidel Castro took control of the Cuban government. The United States endeavored to make a stand through an invasion at the Bay of Pigs, but unfortunately, the strategy was not successful. Because of the unrest in the Caribbean, the United States and the Soviet Union nearly entered into a war with each other. Of concern to the United States and the Allies were Soviet interventions, obvious collaboration, and support of Castro's reign in Cuba. Soon the Soviets invaded eastern Europe, eastern Germany and East Berlin; in order to restrain citizens of that region from leaving, the Berlin Wall was erected, separating East from West for several decades. President John F. Kennedy faced major challenges with the Soviet Union. In another part of the world, the decline of colonial rule in Vietnam attracted worldwide attention as conflict escalated (Brinkley, 2003).

The United States welcomed Hawaii and Alaska as the final states of the union in 1959, forming a federation of 50 states. Despite the positive sentiment surrounding the acquisition of these territories as new states, all was not well within the borders of the United States. Poverty was an issue in several areas of the country, and civil rights were a concern for countless individuals. Antiwar sentiment increased among young adults, civil unrest arose in various locations throughout the United States, and freedom crusades related to social worry intensified. Many citizens took advantage of one of their great freedoms as they voiced concerns and solicited for changes that they felt would stabilize their lives in a time of chaos. President Kennedy, the favorite president of many, was assassinated in 1963, generating speculation of greater Soviet involvement within the United States and even the world. Anticommunist campaigns eventually led to U.S. involvement in both the Korean and Vietnam Wars. The United States was involved in both wars to protect inherent freedoms for those who could not do so effectively.

In 1954, the Supreme Court tried and ruled on *Brown vs. Board of Education* in Topeka, Kansas; the court ruled that racial segregation infringed upon the rights of U.S. citizens and breached the Fourteenth Amendment. Despite this ruling, segregation remained a problem for the next several years. In 1955, Rosa Parks, a Black female, boarded a bus in Alabama and refused to give up her seat in the segregated Black section at the rear of the bus when a White male requested it. She was arrested, and the Black community organized a bus boycott, which invigorated the civil rights movement. A couple of years later in 1957, a high school in Little Rock, Arkansas, became the focus of the nation when several African American students tried to attend an all-White school. President Dwight D. Eisenhower mobilized army soldiers to accompany the students to school and protect them from violence as they entered the school and attended classes (Brinkley, 2003; Kalisch & Kalisch, 2004).

In 1963, Martin Luther King, Jr. delivered his famous "I have a dream" speech. The following year, the Civil Rights Act was introduced and passed as a means to end discrimination. In 1965, the United States bombed North Vietnam; Malcolm X, a Black power leader and civil rights activist, was murdered in New York City; and in 1968, King and his friend, Robert Kennedy, were assassinated in separate incidents (Brinkley, 2003; Mosby, Inc., 2000).

Several other events of interest ultimately influenced medicine and nursing. Antiwar sentiment became a major concern as the Vietnam War escalated and Americans were concerned over great losses and inability of the troops to effect a positive change. During the 1960s, the population of the world surpassed 3 billion, initiating population zero ideology. Polio was almost eradicated in the United States through a national vaccination program. Prior to his assassination, President Kennedy recommended and organized the Peace Corps to encourage world health through personal hygiene and community sanitation programs. Soon after the assassination of President Kennedy, President Lyndon Johnson signed into law the Social Security Act, providing Medicare and Medicaid services to many Americans. The Environmental Protection Agency was organized to safeguard the public, Earth Day was celebrated to increase awareness of caring for the planet, and the use of the pesticide DDT was banned to protect the environment and unborn children. During subsequent years, taking care of the earth became associated with promoting an environment conducive to personal health as well. In the Northeast, many young people attended Woodstock, where they partied and defined views on a number of sensitive issues including the war, drugs, sexual independence, abortion, gender concerns, politics, and segregation. The country was greatly affected by those who proclaimed many new freedoms and rights (Mosby, Inc., 2000).

As President Richard Nixon became associated with Watergate, the Equal Rights Amendment was passed, but not ratified. Nixon resigned before he could be impeached. The Equal Rights Amendment was promoted by feminists and others who supported the cause. IBM and Intel developed computer technology, which accelerated national technology growth and ushered in an age of personal electronics, computer advancements, and eventually the realm of cyberspace and virtual reality. The Twenty-Sixth Amendment was passed in 1971, giving people who were aged 18 or older the right to vote.

Soviet cosmonauts manned the first space flight in 1961, and shortly thereafter, John Glenn was the first American astronaut to orbit the earth through the efforts of the National Aeronautics and Space Administration. Within a decade, men landed on the moon, and the world watched from afar as two Americans explored its surface. The space program accelerated for a number of years, and medical advances that were developed to allow people to live and work in space eventually contributed to medical care and even other aspects of daily living. Some of those innovations are things we now take for granted such as dehydrated food, disposal diapers, physiological monitoring devices, computer technology, satellite communication, and medical research and experimentation on the body related to physics, chemistry, and biology.

The majority of the population lived and often even worked in the suburbs of America. In these communities, many purchased and used goods that previously had been less available to the public, such as automobiles, televisions, and a variety of new modern appliances. McDonald's and other fast food establishments became common places for people to eat, and going to the drive-in movie theater was a popular pastime for many families. Prosperity and economic growth created a larger middle-class America, and the value of capitalism was accepted as the means to eliminate disparity and poverty.

> The nation would simply have to produce more abundance, thus raising the quality of life [for] even the poorest ... to a level of comfort and decency. The right and desire to acquire individual property promoted healthy competition contributing to unprecedented economic growth: a broad consensus about the value and necessity of competitive, capitalistic growth ... [believing] ... in the rights of property, the philosophy of economic individualism, the value of competition; they have accepted the economic virtues of capitalistic culture as necessary. (Brinkley, 2003, 801 and 809)

As families acquired their own television sets, communication innovations brought the world to the people; they were able to observe the Vietnam War, the space missions and moon landing, and everyday news or events in their communities, the nation, and the world. Walt Disney revolutionized entertainment with the *Mickey Mouse Club*, and family programs such as *I Love Lucy, Leave It to Beaver*, and *Ozzie and Harriet* were produced to entertain and characterize the American family of the times. The rock 'n' roll culture initiated during the 1950s became an integral part of life for most youth and young adults; *American Bandstand*, hosted by Dick Clark, helped promote musical artists and their works. Despite greater prosperity for many, there were certain groups who still lived in less than ideal circumstances; one social reformer labeled them "the other America":

> The other America does not contain the adventurous ... it is populated by the failures, by those driven from the land and bewildered by the city, by old people suddenly confronted with the torments of loneliness and poverty, and by minorities facing a wall of prejudice.... [The] invisible land of the other Americans became a ghetto, a modern poor farm, [the elderly] who live out their lives in loneliness and frustration: they sit in rented rooms, or else they stay close to a house in a neighborhood that has completely changed from the old days.... The young are somewhat more visible, yet they too stay close to their neighborhoods. There are tens of thousands of Americans in the big cities who are wearing shoes, perhaps even a stylishly

cut suit or dress, and yet are hungry ... the rejects of society and of the economy ... but they are increasingly isolated from contact with, or sight of, anybody else. Middle-class men and women coming in from Suburbia on a rare trip may catch the merest glimpse of the other America on the way to an evening at the theater, but their children are segregated in suburban schools ... new segregation is compounded by well-meaning ignorance. (Harrington, 1962, 12–13 and 17–18)

The Image of Nursing

FEMALE NURSES OF THE ERA who worked in a hospital or clinic setting wore the traditional white uniform with the symbolic white cap, white hose, white shoes, and, of course, white underwear. Nursing caps reflected educational level. Student nurses wore a plain white cap, associate degree nurses wore a white cap with one stripe on their caps, and baccalaureate degree nurses wore caps with two stripes. Cap styles and shape were specific to the academic or diploma school the nurse attended. Dresses were conservative and had to be below the knee or mid-calf length with short or three-quarter length sleeves generally; some nurses wore wrist-length sleeves. Aprons still used over the dress were most often the symbol of the student nurse. Apprentice nurses wore a variety of solid color dresses with a white pinafore or apron over the top. Female nurses did not wear pants at the beginning of 1960s unless they were associated with military mobile army surgical hospital (MASH) units or certain specialty nursing groups. Surgical scrubs became common in operating room suites, along with a surgical cap and mask. Depending on the circumstances and facility, the females wore scrub dresses and the males wore scrub pants and tops.

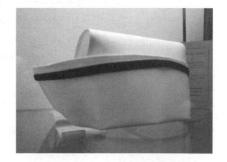

Nurse's cap on display at Seton Medical Center in Daly City, California

Elizabeth Norman commented in an interview on the image of nursing and the subsequent uniform dilemma since the early 1970s. "In the constant struggle for independence from doctors, nurses viewed the white uniform as a symbol of the angelic, demure, dependent woman, not the tough, resourceful professional she really is" (as cited in Houweling, 2004, p. 47). The first part of this symbolic uniform rejected during the late 1960s was the cap; it was cumbersome, no longer even fashionable, and some reported it as a vector for bacteria or other germs in an era where cleanliness was a very important part of all health care. Without their caps, nurses were still identified by their white dresses, white hose, and white shoes; many nurses did wear their caps into the 1980s.

As hospitals transferred purchasing and laundering of the uniform to nurses, they gained a degree of autonomy in deciding what they would wear. Initially those decisions were related to dress styles, and there were some who used equal rights as an opportunity to change the existing rules; soon female nurses were allowed to wear pantsuits to work in many hospitals. One factor that helped to facilitate this change was the presence of more and more male nurses in the hospital. Advanced practice nurses who worked in specialty areas started to replace their white clothing with white labs coats over business attire. During the 1980s, scrubs emerged as the common attire for nurses working in intensive care units, emergency rooms, specialty units, and of course, the surgical areas of the hospital (Houweling, 2004).

Home health nurses still frequently wore a dark colored dress; sometimes they would wear a dark colored suit with a white blouse or even a white dress as their hospital peers did. Most community nurses in the 1960s still wore a traditional nursing cap resembling a cap that might be seen on a hospital nurse. Frontier, rural, or community nurses often put an apron over their clothing to protect themselves and patients when performing certain treatments. Visiting nurses still carried their black bag containing a stethoscope and other patient care supplies. As the era progressed, the length of the dresses shortened to match the style of society. By the end of the 1970s, many community and rural nurses stopped wearing their traditional caps.

War once again influenced the public's perception of nursing; the professional status they had gained attracted naïve nurses into areas of combat. The Vietnam War generated disagreement over the reasons men were sent into combat, but nurses of this war were initially respected by all and revered for the service they rendered under difficult conditions (Mosby, Inc., 2000). Nurses who served in Vietnam went as nurses before them did to care for the war's wounded; many returned with unanticipated wounds of their own despite never having been physically wounded. By the end of the war, military nurses were no longer so venerated; they were "viewed by many as a murderer instead of a healer, [they] felt isolated and angry" (Van Devanter, 1983, inside front dust jacket). Like many other Vietnam veterans ,they suffered from delayed stress syndrome and depression. As they continued to care for hospital patients back in the States, numerous nurses experienced flashbacks and reminders of things they wished to forget. Lynda Van Devanter went to Vietnam to assist in the fight for democracy and came back a changed person. As she counseled women who served in Vietnam as the national women's director of the Vietnam Veterans of America, she reported sleepless nights that came "after reliving Vietnam with another troubled woman veteran" (Van Devanter, 1983, p. 11) who needed support, acceptance, and reassurance.

The Education of Nurses

B Y THE END OF THE 1950s, great importance was placed on an appropriate curriculum and a regimented program to produce a scholarly and well-prepared nurse. The Brown report suggested that nursing schools were responsible for many of the problems associated with nursing education in the United States by midcentury. It found that facilities where nurses were trained were inadequate and in need of improvement. Brown, as cited in Kalisch and Kalisch (2004), recommended in 1948 that there should be a nationwide campaign to improve nursing practice and nursing education. Brown suggested that the following should be considered and addressed:

> Facilities should "be sound in their organizational and financial structure, adequate in facilities and faculty, and well distributed to serve the needs of the entire country." In addition to recommendations related to facilities, the report identified the need for nursing to make "the long overdue official examination of every school" a priority, and requested a list be "published and distributed with a statement to the effect that any school not named had failed to meet the requirements for accreditation." The report called for "a nationwide campaign for the purpose of rallying state boards and non-accredited schools to strong social pressure." It also petitioned for specific "provisions for periodic re-examination of all schools listed" to ensure continued compliance, demanded that "organized nursing commit itself to this undertaking of major social significance," and then requested, "... the public assume responsibility for ... the financial burden. (pp. 132–170)

Schools and nurses responded to the challenge to improve training and to standardize education through mandates supported by the respective state board of nursing. The American Nurses Association (ANA) and the National League for Nursing (NLN) continued to endorse restructuring of nursing education with a focus on each of the educational levels. The consequences of these changes allowed for the formation of "regional assemblies for planning, coordination, and implementation of programs—the councils of Associate Degree Programs, Baccalaureate and Higher Degree Programs, Diploma Programs, Practical Nurse Programs, Hospital and Related Institutional Nursing Services, and Home Health Agencies and Community Health Services" (Donahue, 1996, p. 435).

From 1976 to 1984, the NLN worked to establish and promote educational guidelines in order to define program outcomes and student preparation. In 1984, the NLN advised that nursing research look at education specific for nursing, characteristics of those in nursing, administrative components of nursing, and clinical practice preparation. They issued a credentialing document, *Nursing Roles—Scope and Practice,* which is revised periodically and is a recognized standard for all nursing professionals from a preparation perspective. Since then, additional documents related to scope of practice, educational standards, and mandatory school accreditation for licensure have been introduced by other national nursing organizations. The ANA and NLN promoted the profession as they adopted rigorous standards and expectations for all nurses, and continued to encourage education rather than training so that nurses could use their knowledge wisely, and without routine direction or rote skill implementation. With better theory and improved decision-making capabilities, nurse competency was enhanced and the nurse became "a broker of knowledge" (Huber, 2008).

The ANA initiated a national campaign for certification, especially for advanced practice and specialty nurses. As more of them cared for specific populations, completed higher educational training, participated in research, and developed techniques for best care, a need for recognition of expertise and proficiency became evident. The first of many position papers proposing ideas "to aid the advancement of nursing ... [and] the need for improved nursing practice" (Donahue, 1996, p. 436) was introduced. This document and those that followed defined nursing activity, responsibility, and accountability. As more and more nurses became specialized in the care they provided, specialty nursing organizations arose to address scope of practice, specialty standards, and other issues unique to each domain. These organizations supported the interests of the group without much collaboration with the existing, more generalized professional nursing associations.

In 1966, the following resolution was introduced:

> The education for all those who are licensed to practice nursing should take place in institutions of higher education; minimum preparation for beginning professional nursing practice should be a baccalaureate degree; minimum preparation for a beginning technical nursing practice should be an associate degree in nursing; education for assistants in health service occupations should be short, intensive programs in vocational education rather than on-the-job training. (American Nurses Association's First Position, 1965, p.106)

Loretta Ford, along with a medical peer, introduced a nurse practitioner program in 1965, when primary care physicians could not care for all those who needed access to medical services. Nursing authority was interpreted in new ways as nurses were trained to be nurse practitioners (NP) and clinical nurse specialists (CNS). The emergence of these professionals who were capable of managing patients and other nurses more effectively influenced health care in unanticipated ways and utilized nursing resources as never before imagined. The introduction of NPs and CNSs allowed for nurses to practice much more autonomously as they accepted greater responsibility and authority. Collaboration was necessary in order for doctors and nurses to accomplish best patient care while working together rather than independently. As one of the first pediatric nurse practitioners, Ford felt that promotion of advanced practice roles was ingenious and very significant forsolving social and health problems for specific populations nationally. She promoted the role of the nurse practitioner vigorously for many years. Her efforts were not unlike those of the nurse leaders at the beginning of the 20th century who believed that the health of women and children was a social responsibility (Ford, 1992, pp. 287–297).

Advances in Practice

NURSING WAS AFFECTED BY THE rapid development of the health-care service industry as a result of war, medical advancement, hospital development, and major economic growth. During the later part of the 1950s, the number of health service employees grew by 54%, making health care the third largest industry in the country (Kalisch & Kalisch, 2004). Health care continues to generate a significant amount of revenue today, and it provides more than 16% of the nation's gross national product. U.S. involvement in wars abroad encouraged research, medical techniques, and innovations aimed at altering the medical outcomes for military personnel who experienced traumatic, difficult, or life-threatening conditions. Advancing technology promoted best healthcare practices for them, expanding medical expertise and initiating an age of specialty care areas including coronary care, dialysis, surgical and medical intensive care, oncology, anesthesiology, surgical specialization, burns, and trauma. The demand for health services increased in both civilian and military situations as specific technical care was more readily available. The number of hospitalizations in general increased, as did the cost associated with specialty encounters. As individuals were cared for in the hospital, the majority of them no longer paid for their care by the treatment or for one illness at a time. When they were hospitalized, insurance plans paid for needed services and treatments for almost any condition (Donahue, 1996; Kalisch & Kalisch, 2004).

Focus was on perfecting the care and techniques associated with recent biomedical research in a number of different scientific endeavors. Utilizing scientific advances to promote surprising medical innovations, medical care changed forever. During the 1970s, new and innovative medical techniques modified outcomes and alleviated suffering in areas such as coronary bypass, cardiovascular disease, radiology imaging, renal failure, renal transplants, hemodialysis, artery grafts, fracture plating, chemotherapeutic agents, pharmacology, prosthetic valves of the heart, joint replacements, and microsurgery in neurology and cardiology. Better understanding of pathophysiology in general led to major improvements in the management of many common diseases, most of which in years past caused morbidity and mortality in those affected by them. Vaccines eliminated common infectious diseases, while improved comprehension of cellular biology, physiologic processes, and immunology allowed for rapid expansion of services where nurses and doctors intervened regularly to change the effects of biological processes and ailments.

The motivation and focus of medicine since the turn of the century had been on finding cures for diseases, and the body was often viewed as an object that could be fixed by healthcare providers if they knew what to do and when to do it. With rapid development of technology and its application to patient care during the last 40 years of the century, cost became a variable that was often ignored as cures or improved health were realized. The belief that any cure was best, no matter what the cost if a positive outcome was expected, directed most aspects of individual patient management. This changed when cost containment became a major focus for hospitals and insurance providers limited patient options and provider autonomy.

In the midst of this ideology, Dr. Henry Silverman and Dr. Loretta Ford, a public health nurse, worked together to establish and promote NPs for primary pediatric care and preventive pediatric services. The program was initiated at the University of Colorado and health care was soon revolutionized as NPs were trained to care for patients not only in the ambulatory pediatric setting but also in adult clinics as well. Their focus and care was not unlike that of Lillian Wald, Margaret Sanger, or Mary Brewster in urban settings or the frontier nurses who worked along side Mary Breckinridge, caring for individuals with a variety of illnesses while promoting health for patients and their families. The NP treated patients in a primary care setting as they utilized assessment skills, interpreted diagnostic or laboratory tests, diagnosed common chronic and acute care needs, managed ongoing illness, educated patients, and prescribed or ordered mediations and other treatments. NPs practiced autonomously in many communities, imparting health care to those who often would not otherwise receive routine medical care or preventive services. In many instances, despite great outcomes and interventions to those who were not able to access care easily, physicians and even other nurse peers did not readily accept or recognize their contributions.

The United States Department of Health, Education, and Welfare asserted in a report entitled *Extending the Scope of Nursing Practice* (1972) that

> despite widespread agreement among health professionals that the scope of practice should be extended, there was no consensus about how to do this ... it would be naïve to gloss over the fact that working relationships between physicians and nurses are often less than ideal ... with results that are disadvantageous to both professions ... real and imaginary legal restrictions of nursing practice can be dealt with, and impediments to the extension of nursing can be overcome. (pp. 3–5)

If nurses could expand their services, access to health care for all might be accomplished. The intent of advanced practice roles was not one of competition but one of collaboration because nurses provided primary care to many individuals and families who would not otherwise receive that care.

NPs proved their value in the coming years as they managed and cared for patients in outpatient clinics, rural communities, occupational settings, health maintenance organizations, health departments, and other practice settings. Their success allowed other nurses who trained as CNSs to gain autonomy in the hospital setting, where they managed clinical settings, trained and supervised staff nurses, and directed best overall evidence-based interventions and protocols for their patients. They worked with administrators and physicians to care for patients while they instituted programs to promote best outcomes in an ever-changing healthcare environment.

War and Its Effects on Nursing

IN 1963, MILITARY INVOLVEMENT IN VIETNAM escalated, creating a great need for armed forces nurses. Due to the shortage of nurses nationally, recruitment was difficult, and eventually there were many incentives or bonuses offered to attract them into military service. As the number of military nurses diminished, student financial aid opportunities were enhanced; while nurse trainees were in school, all of their expenses were covered, and most received a salary as well. Vietnam nurses enlisted for a variety of reasons; they volunteered to do great things, including participating in advancing healthcare technology under more dramatic and unique combat

experiences than their predecessors. Just before graduation, these nurses applied for a commission into the
military nurse corps reserves and petitioned for a state
licensing exam. Once they were granted state licensure,
their reserve status changed to that of active duty; soon
they were serving as military nurses either in Asia or
stateside in military facilities. During the war, more than
7,500 nurses served in one of the nurse corps after completing training programs in a civilian hospital or school
(Kalisch & Kalisch, 2004).

The Army Institute of Nursing was created at
Walter Reed Army Hospital under the direction of the
Department of Defense in order to increase the number
of nurses with degrees and encourage reenlistment. In
1966, there were about 200 nurses serving in Vietnam;
by the end of the decade, there were almost 900 military
nurses providing care in a war zone where more Americans had been killed than their enemy. Four nurses who
were injured during the conflict on Vietnamese soil

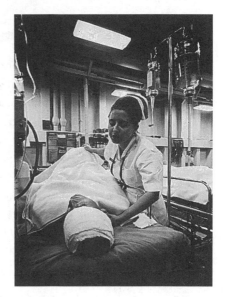

Nurse tends to a patient
on the hospital ship USS
Repose near Vietnam,
1967

received the Purple Heart—the first females to receive such an award. A
congressional bill passed during the war allowed male nurses to be commissioned for regular duty in any service of the armed forces, and within
a year, male nurses accounted for 22% of all of the army's nurses. Many of
these male military nurses worked in specialty areas that were prevalent
in nursing and medical settings (National Advisory Commission on Health
Manpower, 1967).

Unlike nurses during World War II or the Korean Conflict, the nurses
of the Vietnam era were not adequately prepared for the rigors of the war in
which they were eventually involved.

> It was impossible to tell us what we would see, how we were going to feel
> and how much impact it would have on our lives … We realized it was all
> up to us. No one was coming around to tell us what to do … nurses quickly
> learned to assess, to do, and move on … decisions made and actions taken
> were nothing like the civilian nursing world we came from … We triaged
> and proceeded to intubate, insert chest tubes, amputate limbs, and do what-
> ever else was required for our patient's survival … There were no bad nurses

in Vietnam. Our role was much bigger than our training … but being nurses [we] did it well. (Mosby, Inc., 2000, p. 101)

Nurses were initiated into duty almost the moment they arrived in the field; they learned about coping and aspects of survival that were very different from those in the civilian world they had just left. Nurses found it very difficult to live in a war zone; the nurses' daily routine was determined by the surgical and hospital needs, and the war itself dictated daily schedules and activities (Van Devanter, 1983). Due to the fact that most nurses were scheduled to work 12-hour shifts, they were often exhausted. Sleep came after significant exhaustion, and nurses would fall asleep on the dining tables, on the floor, or on chairs pulled together in between cases. Van Devanter describes her experiences:

> With constant patient arrivals we always had someone to care for. [There were] just a lot of things coincidentally happening at the same time … it's a chopper crash, next day a bus accident. Then a mine explodes in a convoy or something else … Plus, there are always the guys who are wounded in battle. It's now 10:30 p.m. and I've been scrubbed since 7 a.m. There are still two operating rooms running. I just hope we don't have to get up again … Let them call somebody else, I have cases scheduled in the morning and don't know how many causalities will come in … It's depressing and yet it's almost reassuring [this routine of ours]. (Van Devanter, 1983, pp. 100, 134–135, 139)

Relationships developed to provide comfort under very difficult circumstances; nurses needed "love, understanding, friendship, and companionship: the things that would keep [them] human in spite of all the inhumanity being practiced around [them]" (Van Devanter, 1983, p. 109). Escape was found in many things, including drugs and alcohol to "block out the faces and the moans of dying boys" (Van Devanter, 1983, p. 108). Nurses were regularly protected by unofficial social directors who made sure the "merrymaking didn't get out of hand ….[Alcohol, and marijuana] packaged like regular cigarettes helped them deal with aspects of living daily in a war zone" (Van DeVanter, 1983, p. 109).

During the war, hospitals and clinics became fixed units instead of just the mobile units used during previous wars. Hospitals were set up in Vietnam and in other countries where rapid response and follow-up care were readily available to the wounded soldiers and civilians. Despite significant injury and illness, about 90% of the soldiers cared for in Vietnam returned to duty as quickly as they could be treated and released. The Veterans Administration became involved with these war veterans because more than 300,000 returned to the United States after the war with disabilities, posttraumatic stress conditions, and major readjustment problems. This was the first war in which so many veterans survived and returned to normal civilian life within days of their release from duty. Their arrival back home was wrought with alienation, isolation, and cultural shock, making the transition much more difficult than in prior military encounters (United States Department of Veterans Affairs, 2007a).

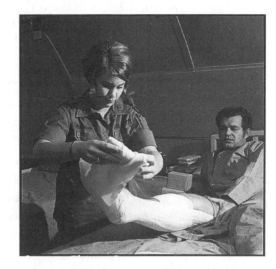

1st Lt. Elaine H. Niggemann changes a surgical dressing for Mr. James J. Torgelson at the 24th Evacuation Hospital, Vietnam, 1971

Congress appropriated funds to deal with medical concerns and the need for ongoing care for these soldiers and nurses. Agent Orange was a chemical that soldiers were exposed to during the conflict. Because of resultant health issues, the Veterans Administration established free ongoing health care to military personnel who experienced illness or a disease not readily identified. The National Academy of Sciences conducted studies and formulated a list of diseases and disabilities that qualified for healthcare benefits, vocational training, and compensation. Many cases of cancer were reported in subsequent years, leading to research and new medical treatments for cancers in general. Spina bifida was also seen in higher incidence among the children of veterans of this war. As more services were required, new facilities emerged to care for those who needed physiological, emotional, and psychological support. Investigations by the National Academy of Sciences contributed much to the body of medical oncology and neurology knowledge in the United States (United States Department of Veterans Affairs, 2007b).

Nursing Workforce Issues

IN THE EARLY 1960s, HEALTH became a major priority for the nation. President Kennedy felt that there was a scarcity of qualified nurses and primary care providers in many areas of the country; he implied that those deficiencies impeded enhancement of national health care. President Johnson agreed that the nursing shortage created a number of concerns for the nation, and during his administration he added Title VIII, the Nurse Training Act of 1964, to the Public Health Service Act, which provided support for the war on poverty and regional medical programs designed to establish opportunities for all related to health care. During this period of time, many interest groups such as the feminists, the Gay Liberationists, the Latinos, the Indians, and the Blacks were demanding equal rights and equal opportunities, including healthcare rights. This act became an extremely important piece of legislation for the future of nursing because it established access to care for all, establishing a pattern for future legislation and funding for nurse interests and education. Changes in nursing roles were directly related to the national goals of health care for all and best standards of practice for any care provided.

The Division of Nursing, part of the Health Resources and Services Administration, in collaboration with the Surgeon General's Consultant Group on Nursing (SGCGN), organized a program that administered nurse training act funds. They promoted the national nursing agenda by consulting, guiding, and evaluating the implementation of the Nurse Training Act. The act recommended that new schools be constructed, that current nursing programs enhance their curriculum, that science become part of all programs, and that nurse educators and facilities study ways to better educate nurses. In order for diploma schools to qualify for federal funds, they had to incorporate guidelines from the National League for Nursing into their program; if they complied with the national guidelines developed by the National League for Nursing and the Association of Collegiate Schools of Nursing, their students were eligible for partial government support. The National League for Nursing worked closely with the Division of Nursing to continue traineeship programs for students who could benefit from low-interest student loans. This act provided funding only to National League for Nursing-accredited schools originally; however, nonaccredited schools eventually received funding if they complied with the NLN standards (United States Congressional Budget Office, 1976, pp. 14 and 35–39).

This legislation was designed to continue preparing nurses for service in the United States and was not passed in relation to any war nursing needs. It was, however, passed to alleviate a registered nurse shortage and to enhance the availability of nurses nationally, especially outside the urban centers. It further increased funding for nurses to enhance their education past the associate degree level. The traineeship bill enhanced the number of minority students who were educated in the basic level nurse training programs. The funding also promoted nursing education for nurses who might work in the community or the outpatient setting. Finally, funds could be used to develop recruitment techniques and campaigns to solicit new nurses (United States Congressional Budget Office, 1976, pp. 35–36 and 41–46).

Despite lack of recognition for nursing services prior to this time, men provided care to soldiers in a number of American military endeavors. During the Revolutionary War, according to Major Charlotte Scott, as quoted in O'Lynn & Tranbarger (2007), there was

> inadequate help in caring for the sick and wounded soldiers during this conflict ... commanders pulled soldiers from the front lines to provide care to those in need. Although these "providers" were not nurses in the formal sense of the word, the need to provide care to the sick and the wounded was clear. (p.84)

During the Civil and Spanish American Wars, male soldiers gave care to wounded comrades on the battlefield. These groups of men were part of the Hospital Corps, which trained certain soldiers specifically for battlefield care; in reality their role was that of an orderly or medic. Working in collaboration with these men were female nurses, some of whom were volunteers and some of whom had training. The surgeon general at the beginning of the 20th century "opposed maintaining female nurses in military facilities, as the corpsmen would not be able to focus on their duties if they had to work side by side with female nurses" (O'Lynn & Tranbarger, 2007, p. 55).

However, the influence of nurse leaders and reformers ultimately influenced Congress and other political leaders such that men were finally able to serve as military nurses by 1955. Prior to that time they could only function in the role of a medic, who worked alongside female nurses that were allowed to care for soldiers and civilians alike. From 1960 to 1980, many males participated in military nursing, benefiting from the work of those who had promoted the cause of the missing male nurse. They eventually found their way into civilian hospitals and nursing units (Kalisch & Kalisch, 1986).

Because of influence from nurse reformers and feminists, men generally were not eligible to apply for admission into established nursing programs in the hospital setting prior to this era. Even within the realm of home health or private duty nursing, men were all but eliminated in many parts of the country from the practice of nursing. Major William Terriberry stated in 1908 that "the lack of male nurses in the United States is due to the lack of demand for them. In hospitals there is a small need for them now, and in the future this need will decrease" (as quoted in Bester, 2007, p. 85). Because of this type of sentiment, many decades passed before male nurses were accepted into the profession.

As nursing services were recognized as a valuable addition to the military, the Army Nurse Corps was established to encourage nursing and to help alleviate a nursing shortage as the need for nurses in both the military and civilian arena increased; one of the limitations of the Army Nurse Corps was that only female nurses were eligible for training and service until the mid-1960s. Even during the two world wars, males could not work as nurses; they could only work as orderlies in army hospitals alongside their female counterparts, who were real nurses. Despite repeated attempts to include them into the Nurse Corps, for the first half of the 20th century they were not commissioned nor allowed to work as registered nurses. Efforts of the ANA eventually helped the cause of males in the nursing profession as it supported them as qualified individuals who met the national standards, fulfilled educational requirements, and satisfied licensure requisites through examination (Bester, 2007).

Licensure and Regulation

LICENSURE BECAME A REQUIREMENT FOR all nurses and was determined by state boards of nursing in collaboration with professional national nursing associations. Each individual nurse was required to complete educational standards in accordance with recommendations by the ANA, the

NLN, and the American Association of Critical Care Nurses. These national councils encouraged collaboration of schools and curriculums through a national board. Eventually they organized and managed test administration for licensure; initially, it was the State Board Test Pool Exam that controlled the administration of nursing exams. By the early 1980s the first National Council Licensure Exam (NCLEX) was given to graduating nurses. The exam became associated with the nurse's ability to practice because obtaining licensure was dependent on achieving a predetermined score. This exam is still used to determine competency of new graduates.

Nursing Research

DURING THE 1960s AND 1970s, the nurse scientist emerged with the development of university and nursing science departments, which studied nursing interventions and cultivated theories specific to the discipline of nursing. Throughout the 1960s, universities were granted funds for interdisciplinary research and training programs in which nurses studied. Funds from the Division of Nursing initially were dispersed mainly at the graduate level during the 1950s; however, doctoral research and even postdoctorate work was encouraged. Legislation at the national level focused on increasing the number of better prepared nurses while improving patient care and outcomes. Funding became available to accomplish this through the Nurse Training Act.

In 1962, the first research field office for the Department of Nursing was opened in San Francisco to examine nursing issues such as staffing and patients' needs, best interventions for diabetes, specialty care concerns, nurse utilization, nurse preceptors and educators, and adequate educational opportunities for nurses. With initiation of this early field office and eventually others, federal resources moved closer to nurse investigators and their research. The SGCGN was formed and commissioned to provide support for nursing research, hospital administration, nursing leaders, and the public. Their major goals were to improve quality of nursing care and to promote programs aimed at decreasing the nursing shortage that began after World War II. Through the efforts of the SGCGN and its recommendations for governmental support, a number of grants and scholarships for nurses, as well as funds to build new schools or improve established nursing schools began to be awarded (United States Congressional Budget Office, 1976, pp. 42–46).

Efforts of the Association of Collegiate Schools of Nursing, Sigma Theta Tau, the ANA, and new government-sponsored programs under the direction of the SGCGN ushered in an era of nursing research and nursing theory. Not all nurses were "fitted for investigation … encouraged by [Isabel] Stewart an increasing number of students did undertake doctoral studies … [as she] laid the foundation for nursing research and research preparation in the Division of Nursing" (McManus, 1962, p. 6). Her efforts initiated funding opportunities for many students through nurse-scientist graduate training programs at the master's and doctorate level in college-affiliated programs. The focus on documentation of nurse activity, nurse interventions and outcomes, and the acquisition of theory specific to nursing validated the profession from 1960 to 1980 and long afterwards.

Nurse activists and reformers since Florence Nightingale changed the way that nurses cared for patients and their roles in the healthcare community. Their ideas and diligence promoting the cause of nursing led others to generate "knowledge and to assist with the definition and identification of the unique role and functions of nursing" (Donahue, 1996, p.421). Nurse researchers and scholars attempted to answer questions such as: What is nursing? What do nurses really do? How do they influence patient care and patient outcomes? What is the value of nursing services? What types of interactions occur? How do nurse–patient relationships affect health and wellness outcomes? Several nurses developed concepts that are often referred to as nursing theories; they described the phenomena of nursing, their knowledge, their interventions, their assessments and analysis, and the creation of their work. These concepts include the following:

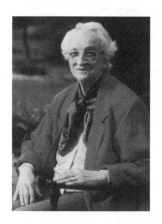

Nursing theorist
Hildegard Peplau

- Hildegard Peplau coined the phrase, *psychodynamic nursing,* to describe the nurse–patient relationship. She identified the following four phases of this relationship: (1) the person and the nurse identify problem(s); (2) needed help is recognized mutually; (3) there is acceptance of reasonable goal(s); and

(4) assistance leads to independence once again. During the relationship the nurse assumes a number of roles as she assists the patient (Peplau, 1952).

- Virginia Henderson (1966) described a nurse's function as an agent:

  to assist the individual (sick or well) in the performance of those activities [promoting] health or its recovery or a peaceful death ... he would perform it unaided if he had the necessary strength, will, or knowledge ... to do this in such a way as to help him gain independence as rapidly as possible. (p. 15)

- Martha Rogers (1970) recognized nursing as a science that is "translated into nursing practice. Only as the science of nursing takes on form and substance can the art of nursing achieve new dimensions" (p. 86). She linked physical abstract science to health and caring.

- One individual who studied Rogers's ideas is Margaret Newman. In 1972, Newman described the relationship between the patient, the nurse, and the environment as:

  a manifestation of an evolving pattern of interaction ... We are in the process of expanding consciousness and sometimes we don't recognize it because we don't recognize the pattern of our lives and we don't recognize it in the process of illness and disease even though it's there ... The important thing is for the nurse to be able to help the person get on with movement in terms of expanding consciousness. (pp. 449–451)

- Imogene King's *General Systems Framework* (1971) emphasized the interactions between the nurse and the patient in relation to the environment.

- Ida J. Orlando's *Nursing Process Theory* (1961) described how nurses cared for patients by using their cognitive skills to assess and implement appropriate care based on the scientific process.

- In 1964, Ernestine Wiedenbach wrote a thesis called *Helping Art of Clinical Nursing*, which defined nursing as an art that is not reactionary, but rather a series of deliberate actions to help the patient achieve equilibrium between optimal health and illness.

- Jean Watson organized 10 carative factors in her 1979 work, *Philosophy and Science of Caring.* These factors were used to describe caring related to person, environment, health, and nursing. She believes that in a society that doesn't know how to value caring, nurses are able to define what caring is and demonstrate that it is actually an art and a science.

- Dorothea Orem's *Self-Care Deficit Theory of Nursing* (1959) defined nursing as necessary to sustaining life and health when patients are unable to do that for themselves. The model describes how a nurse helps the patient return to the optimum level of self-care.

- In the mid-1970s, Betty Neuman proposed her systems model, which explained an individual's reaction to health and wellness as an attempt to achieve equilibrium in the dynamic state of nature by balancing physiological, spiritual, emotional, psychological, and cultural aspects of life.

Summary

THE UNITED STATES EXPERIENCED a number of internal issues related to freedom. Liberation of youth, segregation, and gender were all topics that were associated with an equal rights agenda. Media influence contributed to successes of those who were seeking equality; however, it brought into the daily lives of people aspects of daily living that had not been so obvious prior to 1960. The Vietnam War, space flights, Woodstock, civil unrest, and national politics were distressing to many who before had lived their lives in bliss. Innovations and advances associated with the space programs and computer technology encouraged many changes in medical care. Specialty services became an area of focus, and hospitalizations increased significantly.

The Brown report forced nurses to look at education and to reevaluate the process. Collaborative relationships among colleges and universities allowed for national standards to be defined, for educational levels to be evaluated, for licensure and certification to be refined, and for scope of practice to be outlined. National nursing organizations explained specific scopes of practice in order for state licensing boards to regulate practice. Feminism and equality once again affected nursing; some consequences of integration allowed for male nurses to be more involved in the nursing profession and for minority nurses to gain a national nursing presence. Specialization encouraged male nurses to become involved in technical and acute care nurse settings.

❧ IDEAS FOR FURTHER EXPLORATION

1. Learn more about nursing theorists and their work to describe and validate nursing. Compile a summary list of three to five theorists and the basic premises of their work.
2. Choose an area of biomedical research that interests you and briefly share how it affects nursing care or specialty care today. Remember computer and space technology. List three to five of those accomplishments and describe how they influenced nursing care.
3. What effect did the Brown report have on nursing? What things did it change? Did those changes influence nursing in the future? How?

⯎ DISCUSSION QUESTIONS: APPLICATION TO CURRENT PRACTICE

1. What affect did the equal rights and/or the feminist movement have on nursing? Are there implications for practice today because of those effects? Choose two or three topics to describe and discuss.
2. From 1960 to the early 1980s, educational competency became a concern. How did nursing practice change as competency was addressed? Did advanced practice roles change this? Why or why not? Explain how nursing theory and competency are related. Give specific examples.
3. The National Council Licensure Exam was accepted as the examination for all graduate nurses. How did it change practice? Does its influence determine nursing licensure or credentialing today? Give examples and relate them to scope of practice and competency.

⯎ MeSH SEARCH TERMS

Credentialing	Education, nursing, graduate
Education, nursing, associate	Nursing research
Education, nursing, baccalaureate	Vietnam Conflict

Other useful non-MeSH search terms:

National Council Licensure Exam	Army Institute of Nursing
Brown report	

◆ SUGGESTED READING

Freedman, D., & Rhoads, J. (1987). *Nurses in Vietnam: The forgotten veterans*. Austin, TX: Texas Monthly Press.

Hampton, L. (1992). *The fighting strength: Memoirs of a combat nurse in Vietnam*. New York: Warner Books.

Keeling, A. W. (2007). *Nursing and the privilege of prescription, 1893–2000*. Columbus: Ohio State University Press.

Norman, E. M. (1990). *Women at war: The story of fifty military nurses who served in Vietnam*. Philadelphia: University of Pennsylvania Press.

Stanton, J. (2002). *Innovations in health and medicine: Diffusion and resistance in the twentieth century*. London: Routledge.

Stapleton, D. H., Welch, C. A., & the Foundation of the New York State Nurses Association. (1994). *Critical issues in American nursing in the twentieth century: Perspectives and case studies*. Guilderland, NY: The Foundation.

◆ REFERENCES

American Nurses Association's first position on education for nursing. (1965). *American Journal of Nursing, 65*(12), 106–111.

Bester, W. T. (2007). Army nursing: A personal biography. In C. E. O'Lynn & R. E. Tranbarger (Eds.), *Men in nursing: History, challenges, and opportunities* (pp. 83–98). New York: Springer.

Brinkley, A. (2003). *American history: A survey* (11th ed.). New York: McGraw-Hill.

Donahue, M. P. (1996). *Nursing: The finest art* (2nd ed.). St. Louis, MO: Mosby.

Ford, L. C. (1992). Advanced nursing practice: Future of the nurse practitioner. In L. H. Aiken, . & C. M. Fagin (Eds.), *Charting nursing's future: Agenda for the 1990s*. Philadelphia: J.B. Lippincott.

Harrington, M. (1962). *The other American*. New York: Macmillan Publishing Co.

Henderson, V. (1966). *The nature of nursing: A definition and its implications for practice, research, and education*. New York: Macmillan.

Houweling, L. (2004). Image, function, and style: A history of the nursing uniform. *American Journal of Nursing, 104*(4), 40–48.

Huber, D. (2008, August 19). Personal communication.

Kalisch, P. A., & Kalisch, B. J. (1986). *The advance of American nursing* (2nd ed.). Boston: Little, Brown.

Kalisch, P. A., & Kalisch, B. J. (2004). *American nursing: A history* (4th ed). Philadelphia: Lippincott, Williams, and Wilkins.

McManus, R. L. (1962). Isabel M. Stewart—Foremost researcher. *Nursing Research, 2*, 6.

Mosby, Inc. (2000). *Nursing reflections: A century of caring*. St. Louis, MO: Mosby.

National Advisory Commission on Health Manpower. (1967). *Report of the National Advisory Commission on Health Manpower, Vol. 1*. Washington, DC: Government Printing Office.

Newman, M. A. (1972). Nursing's theoretical evolution. *Nursing Outlook, 20*(7), 449–453.

O'Lynn, C. E., & Tranbarger, R. E. (2007). *Men in nursing: History, challenges, and Opportunities*. New York: Springer.

Peplau, H. E. (1952). *Interpersonal relations in nursing, a conceptual frame of reference for psychodynamic nursing*. New York: Putnam.

Rogers, M. E. (1970). *An introduction to the theoretical basis of nursing.* Philadelphia: F. A. Davis Co.

United States Congressional Budget Office. (1976). *Nursing education and training: Alternative federal approaches.* Congress of the United States. Retrieved August 28, 2008, from http://www.cbo.gov/ftpdocs/67xx/doc6711/78-CBO-003.pdf

United States Department of Health, Education, and Welfare, Secretary's Committee to Study Extended Roles of Nurses. (1972). *Extending the scope of nursing practice: A report of the Secretary's committee.* Washington, DC: Government Printing Office.

United States Department of Veterans Affairs. (2007a). *America's wars fact sheet.* Washington, DC: Office of Public Affairs.

United States Department of Veterans Affairs. (2007b). *VA history in brief.* Retrieved August 10, 2008, from http://www1.va.gov/opa/feature/history/index.asp

Van Devanter, L. (with Morgan, C.). (1983). *Home before morning: The story of an Army nurse in Vietnam.* New York: Beaufort Books.

Watson, J. (1979). *Nursing: The philosophy and science of caring.* Boston: Little, Brown.

Wiedenbach, E. (1964). *Clinical nursing, a helping art.* New York: Springer.

CHAPTER 9

Nursing in the United States
From the 1980s to the Present

Early 1980s Diagnosis-related groups (DRGs) established

1980–2008 · Advancement in nursing knowledge and theory
· Scientific and technological endeavors advance healthcare opportunities

1998
Tobacco Master Settlement Agreement funds help reduce smoking and defray medical costs

1986
Chernobyl nuclear accident

1989
Fall of Berlin Wall

1980	1982	1984	1986	1988	1990	1992	1994	1996	1998

1981
AIDS identified

1987
DNA first used to convict criminals

1991
· Soviet Union collapse
· Cold War ends

1995
Ebola virus spreads in Zaire

1996
Dolly, the first cloned sheep, is born

1990–1991 Persian Gulf War

1990–2000 Nurse practitioner roles differentiated

1990–2008 · Right to die issues and limitation of health services explored
· Outpatient surgery/specialty clinics replace traditional hospital services
· Cost containment and reform

1995–2008 Home health services improve, resurgence of home health care

NEW OPPORTUNITY, TECHNOLOGICAL ADVANCES, NURSING AUTONOMY AND GLOBALIZATION

Deborah M. Judd

2000–2008 Nursing organizations restructure

2002–2008 Expansion of palliative care and hospice services

2005–Present Obesity epidemic

2006–2008 Historical presidential campaign involves minority candidates

2000	2001	2002	2003	2004	2005	2006	2007	2008

2000
- Preventative health care promoted
- 5% of nurses are male & 12% are other minorities
- 9/11 terrorist attacks
- War in Afghanistan begins

2003
- Center for American Nurses founded to promote healthy work environments
- Iraq War begins

2005
Doctor of nursing practice (DNP) programs started

2008
- U.S. economic crisis and bailout
- Barack Obama elected president

OUR NURSING HERITAGE: KEY PEOPLE

The work of nurse theorists and researchers continued into this period and still continues to this day. There really are too many individual nurses contributing to the practice of nursing now to mention them all by name.

The following organizations or associations are changing nursing heritage. Member nurses or other groups of nurses throughout the nation contribute to the body of knowledge for nurses. Their collective efforts have defined or are defining nursing practice.

American Nurses Association (ANA)

National League for Nursing (NLN)

International Council of Nurses (ICN)

American Nurses Credentialing Center (ANCC)

American Association of Colleges of Nursing (AACN)

National Council of State Boards of Nursing (NCSBN)

Specialty practice organizations (a variety of them address special nursing interest)

Advanced practice organizations

Administrative/information technology organizations

Educational organizations

Legal nurse and consulting organizations

State and regional associations

Hattie M. Bessant	First Black nurse researcher to receive a grant for mental health studies
	Supported minority nurse roles
	Encouraged access to care for all
Madeleine Leninger	Nurse researcher and theorist
	Transcultural Competence Model
Nola Pender	Nurse researcher and theorist
	Health Promotion Model
Patricia Benner	Nurse researcher and theorist
	From Novice to Expert

Sociopolitical Climate

A S THE 1970S CONCLUDED, MANY Americans had great reservations about the ability of the national government to manage the country as a whole. Although segregation became less problematic and Vietnam and Watergate were almost forgotten, the presidents who followed Richard Nixon faced great challenges internally as well as externally. Human rights became a concern as the country moved from more self-serving relationships outside the United States to a diplomacy program that promoted traditional freedoms for all. President Jimmy Carter negotiated the return of the Panama Canal as he arbitrated a final treaty between Israel and Egypt in the Middle East. However, as this treaty was negotiated and signed, American hostages were taken in Iran and the Soviets invaded Afghanistan while the nation dealt with an extraordinary energy crisis.

Soviet activity caused the world to take note when the United States, along with other nations, boycotted the Olympics in Moscow. Several other international events, such as the Soviet presence in Poland, the Nicaraguan revolution, the Israel/Lebanon conflict, Soviet leadership changes, terrorist attacks in Beirut, the Iran hostility, Chinese student rebellions, and changes in South African apartheid caused all nations a certain degree of uneasiness. With changes in the Soviet government and a more global awareness of deserved freedoms, the Berlin Wall was broken down to reunite Germany, and the Eastern European states attained independence from Communist rule. Americans and many others throughout the world rejoiced because they believed the Cold War had ended. Despite the realization of self-regulation in many of these countries, great unrest, oppression, and human suffering followed as they determined how they would be governed and how they would deal with the associated issues of that process (Brinkley, 2003).

In the United States, a more conservative pattern of social and economic growth emerged during the Ronald Reagan years, as a progressive world economy added to opportunities and problems within the nation. A recession, the worst since the Great Depression, was associated with previous national and international sociopolitical events, including the worldwide energy crisis. Policies were developed to reclaim the economy through control of taxation, government spending, and specific regulations on the Federal Reserve. Despite positive intentions, the cost of entitlement programs such as Social

Security, Medicare, Medicaid, welfare assistance, student loans, school lunch programs, state federal assistance initiatives, and increased military spending exceeded the effect of budget restraints. President George H. W. Bush took office in 1989 and the Democratic Congress made little progress related to domestic issues. Armament agreements were pursued with the Soviets, and the economy continued to recover gradually through a series of severe budget constraints; however, the process was slow and eventually forced some individuals and businesses to declare bankruptcy, causing concern for many. Considerable debate over military spending followed since the Soviet bloc, once a major threat to world peace, was no longer that. Despite a movement to decrease military resources and spending, supported even by the president, the administration ordered an invasion of Panama and eventually Iraq and Kuwait as the United States continued to "use its power actively not to fight communism, but to defend regional economic interests" (Brinkley, 2003, p. 913) from leaders who would use their power unwisely and threaten goals of worldwide peace and global cooperation.

The nation had emerged as a global leader, an international arbitrator, and peacemaker. However, on September 11, 2001, all Americans stopped and faced the tragic news that four American planes had been hijacked by Islamic terrorists. Three of the planes were crashed into their intended targets (the World Trade Center and the Pentagon), but one of the four crashes did not happen as was planned due to the interventions of the plane's passengers and crew, who forced the plane down prior to reaching the intended target. "There was one great continuity between the world of the 1990s and the world that began on September eleventh.... The United States was becoming deeply entwined in a new age of globalism," (Brinkley, 2003, p. 919) which came with many promises, but also the possibility of great peril.

The Image of Nursing

COMPLEXITY OF HEALTH CARE, NURSING autonomy, advanced practitioners, nurse administrators, nurse educators, nurse politicians, the universal scrub, and the changing character of the nation transformed the face of the nurse. Minority nurses practice alongside male nurses and the white female nurse in a variety of settings and roles. Furthermore, the nurse might be a veteran, baby boomer nurse, or he or she might be a member of Generation X or Y—a "nexter," or a "millennial." An influx of medical professionals from other countries have affected the face of nursing as well.

When nurses readily adopted the scrub uniform as their universal attire for clinical and hospital settings, the ability to determine what they would wear became more of an issue of individual expression. Some selected clothing adorned with a variety of cartoons or other patterned fabrics, while others decided upon the solid-colored scrubs available in a wide range of colors. Individual preferences were satisfied as scrub companies stylized the uniform and introduced new fabrics.

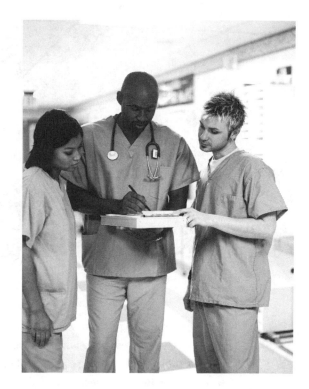

> [Nurses] think nothing of wearing clothing adorned with cartoon characters. What other professions that serve the public have cartoon characters on their uniform? Police officers, hospital staff, judges, firefighters, and others would not be seen with Snoopy, Sponge Bob [sic], or animal characters covering their uniform... No wonder you have no authority. (Cohen, 2007, p. 25)

Nursing has been rated the most honest profession since the beginning of the millennium, but is this truly its image? Nurses want and need to look like the professionals they desire to be. Today, patients, family members, and other healthcare providers do not know who the nurse is by his or her apparel. One might say that the demeanor and presentation of a nurse might help distinguish who she is; but if you are sick and hospitalized or if you are a family member of someone who needs help under less than ideal circumstances, can you discern the professional nurse that way? White uniforms are no longer the symbol that nurses wear daily, "but there is no question that identity is crucial and that everyone needs to be able to recognize the nurse" (Houweling, 2004).

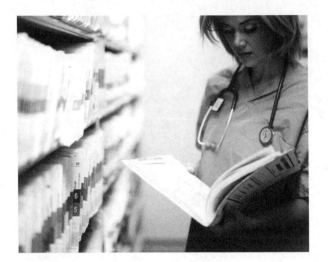

Cohen (2007) suggested that nurses' image will require a nurturing process in this century. As they define who they really are, they will need to (1) show that they value nursing and prove that image daily; (2) take themselves seriously and dress the part; (3) recognize the merit of what they do; and (4) believe they and their peers are professionals (p. 25). Changes in health care have ushered in an era of cost containment and efficiency of services. Within any organization, that has translated into utilization of the least number of nurses to perform required patient care. Does the uniform quandary hide the fact that nurses may or may not be present? In the eyes of those who receive care, nurses do not appear any different from the certified nurse assistant, the medical assistant, the medical assistant certified, the respiratory therapist, the dietician, the surgical scrub or tech, or any number of other allied health providers. They may not even appear different from the physician, physician assistant, or nurse practitioner who wears scrubs during certain procedures. Many of these providers cover their scrubs with a traditional white lab coat, which might distinguish them from the rest of those who wear the utilitarian scrub.

Nurses' image is not only dependent on what they wear, it is based on how they act in or out of the workplace and on the care they provide for those in their charge. Appropriate behavior, best interpersonal relationships, collaboration with peers, proper management of patients, and adequate mentoring and support of nursing peers will do much to support the image they desire. Nurses can identify themselves and state:

> "I am _____, your registered nurse. I am working with _____. She/he is your nurse assistant. I will take care of you today, so let me know if you need anything."

Nurses might also inform patients of what they are doing for them as they interact with them; for example, "This is your blood pressure medicine. I will check later to make sure that it is working, and if it is not doing what it is supposed to do, I will work with your doctor to make sure that you get what you need." This scripting allows patients to know that the nurse is in charge of their care and will be working collaboratively with their medical provider.

As nurses work together to support the profession, they will be able to help the public, their peers, their employers, and themselves understand better that nurses are professionals with an identity and mission that is unique to them. Protecting their image is important. "The irony is clear; nursing dress has gone from being entirely unregulated [during the mid- to late 1800s] to being extremely regimented [hospital, diploma, and university standards], to being back nearly where we started" (Houweling, 2004, p. 48). Nurses' behavior away from work will determine what their future image may be. "If we roll our eyes and complain about the day, what message have we sent about our profession?" (Cohen, 2007, p. 25). If nurses tell their children and others that they don't want them to become nurses for reasons such as nurses not being respected, nurses being underpaid, people having unrealistic expectations of nurses, or nurses not being valued by administration, then what are the implications professionally, if any?

The Education of Nurses

NURSING HAS DEBATED TWO QUESTIONS related to education for almost 50 years. First, what should the entry level education be for practice as a registered nurse—associate or baccalaureate? Secondly, should all nurses be required to participate in continuing education as part of active or inactive practice? The percentage of nurses practicing with a variety of educational degrees or diplomas has fluctuated greatly; until the 1960s, most nurses were diploma nurses, and their education was provided by a hospital or hospital school, not a college or university.

Table 9-1 compares aspects of associate and baccalaureate education.

TABLE 9-1　Aspects of Associate and Baccalaureate Education

Concept	Associate Preparation: Associate Degree in Nursing (ADN)	Baccalaureate Preparation: Bachelor of Science in Nursing (BSN)
Nursing care: Patient Significant others	Direct care administered by involves common, simple, and defined interventions and diagnoses.	Direct care administered involves a more complex nursing process, including multiple nursing diagnoses and interventions, individualized care plans, and greater initiative characteristics.
Practice structure	Require defined, specific protocols and procedures to follow; their limited theoretical knowledge decreases independent decision making and diagnostic ability.	Can work more autonomously and without as many defined protocols and procedures related to nursing judgments, planning, decisions, and implementation.
Communication	The patient is the focus of communication; basic therapeutic communication is used, primarily with peers.	Can act as patient advocates and are in charge of the complex web of communication that involves the patient and other multidisciplinary team members.
Patient education	Can use standardized materials and plans for patient education.	Can identify a need for and tailor patient education, devising individualized strategies or concepts.
Nursing research	Understand that research influences practice and can access standardized information, but contribute little data collection.	Participate in research related to aspects of care, can initiate new ideas based on evidence-based practice, and can collaborate on ideas and resources.
Organization and management	Can organize and manage care of patients, including interaction with significant others.	Can organize a complex process of management related to patient responsibility, setting, and management of other peers.

Concept	Associate Preparation: Associate Degree in Nursing (ADN)	Baccalaureate Preparation: Bachelor of Science in Nursing (BSN)
Accountability	Responsible for self, for delegation to and oversight of licensed practical nurses, licensed vocational nurses, and other unlicensed assistive personnel.	Responsible for self; for delegation of care to peers with equivalent knowledge and skills; for managing and accepting oversight of licensed practical nurses, licensed vocational nurses, or unlicensed assistive personnel; for maintaining education; and for teaching peers.
Nursing care	Care is focused on the overall period of contact (i.e., admission to discharge) and implementation of a focused plan.	Care encompasses the period of contact and extends beyond present, includes follow-up and future treatment plans or educational needs.

Source: Adapted from Hood, L. J., & Leddy, S. K. (2006). *Leddy & Pepper's conceptual bases of professional nursing* (6th ed.). Philadelphia: Lippincott, Williams, & Wilkins.

Professional nursing is based upon acquired knowledge and eventual practiced expertise and experience. There are aspects of professional nursing, however that cannot be acquired through hands-on practice. Research, theory, complex cognitive skills, and leadership are principles that must be taught in the educational arena and then practiced. Because of continued debate over preparation, the entry level of education for practice does not yet have a national standard. Despite the deliberation over basic entry level for practice, diploma programs have decreased from the 1970s to the present. Spratley, Johnson, Sochalski, Fritz, and Spencer (2001) reported that only 60 diploma hospital programs remain in the entire country, a decrease from over 2,500 programs during the 1920s. These programs have incorporated science and social instruction into the nursing curriculum in order to meet National League for Nursing (NLN) standards for accreditation. Even if a school was not accredited, nurses could take the licensure exam if the schools met national curriculum patterns. Nurses at the time of this research conducted by Spratley et al. worked with the following educational degrees:

- Associate's degree—34%

- Baccalaureate degree—31%

- Master's degree or a PhD degree—10%

- Diploma or associate degree—one third of all students seeking a baccalaureate degree, yet these students accounted for less than 3% of all nurses who did not hold the baccalaureate degree

- Associate's degree, in the process of obtaining the baccalaureate degree— 16%

Associate degree programs created to deal with the nursing shortage during the 1950s prepared most entry level nurses—about 60% of them. The Nurse Training Act of 1985 provided federal funding once again to assist nurses in their quest for education as they acquired knowledge and skills to provide the best evidence-based practice to the nation. The Division of Nursing recommended that these federal funds be used primarily for graduate programs to promote and expand the roles of NPs, CNSs, and other certified nurses. Many nurses participated in specialty certifications offered through professional organizations with additional hands-on or theory experience required in the area of certification. Professional educational standards were reviewed; it was felt that certification programs should be shifted into academic programs where nurses would complete a master's degree program and become eligible for licensure and certification at the national level. Nurse practitioner programs throughout the nation adopted this approach to education by the end of the 20th century. Over time, nurse practitioner programs—originally more common to either an adult population or a pediatric population—developed specialty focus areas, changing educational programs and graduate preparation to meet the needs of the nation.

Preparation of nurses today focuses on utilization of the nursing process, acquisition of scientific or evidence-based practices and standards, application of nursing research into the clinical realm, theory and practice of clinical skills, and an understanding of cultural, social, emotional, physiological, and psychological aspects of caring. Nurse educators are responsible for facilitating learning so that students can function independently as they use practical technical skills and cognitive skills for appropriate decision making and nursing interventions. All nurses are now held to very specific standards of practice, which have been defined by the American Association of Nurses and other specialty organizations. Students learn the basics of practice at the associate degree level and then are required to further their knowledge through direct patient care, further academic studies, courses focused on specialty areas of nursing, organization-based in-service or facility programs, and other types of training or certification. The NLN, the American Association of Colleges of Nursing, and the Commission on Collegiate Education continue to regulate nursing education requirements so that graduate nurses are ready to take their nursing board examination.

The experience of the nursing student is no longer what it was a few years ago. Significant time and effort are still required to attain all the technical and theoretical skills necessary for students to graduate and be prepared for the national nursing test, the National Council for Nursing Licensure Examination, which assesses competency and allows nurses to be licensed in the state of their choice once they have passed the exam. Great emphasis is placed on cognitive skills and the ability to use what the student has learned in applicable ways for best patient care. Decision making is crucial for a well-prepared nurse and is the result of practice in the clinical setting.

A significant number of clinical hours are still needed for completion of any undergraduate program. During the first 2 years of the actual nursing courses, students spend considerable time completing their clinical rotations. As was the case 100 years ago, students still feel that an inordinate amount of time is spent in perfecting technical skills. Today, however, there are new educational opportunities for practical experiences. Simulation and computer technology allow for students to perform and practice necessary skills in a laboratory setting or on the computer through virtual reality encounters. Books and other reference materials are readily available in print or online, giving students the ability to learn in new and exciting ways.

Discussion began early in the 21st century about the Doctorate of Nursing Practice (DNP). It involved a change in educational preparation for all advanced practice nurses to that of doctorate rather than master's degree. The Commission on Collegiate Education, the accrediting body of the American Association of Colleges of Nursing, determined in 2005 that only programs with a practice doctorate degree using the credential DNP would be considered by their organization for accreditation. This new degree allowed for enhancement of the profession, improvement of nursing practice, strengthened evidence-based patient outcomes, and defined competency of advanced practice nursing. "Clinicians demonstrate integrative and holistic thinking patterns, while researchers tend to be reductionists in their thought processes" (Apold, 2008, p. 103). A DNP will represent competency in a number of areas relevant to clinical practice. Educators continue "to include a variety of advanced skills such as information systems and technology, healthcare policy development, advanced epidemiology, and prevention strategies" in programs that are already filled with many clinical hours and much theory (Apold, 2008, p. 103).

Since there is a wide range of expertise associated with specific clinical roles at the PhD level, it was believed that clinicians should be identified differently than their peers the nurse researcher and the nurse educator. Master's degree nursing programs usually require more graduate credits than other healthcare disciplines do. The DNP would be comparable to other doctoral degrees and permit nurses who devote time to advanced practice degrees to have a more comparable use of time and resources.

Advances in Practice

NEARLY A CENTURY AGO families cared for their ill and infirm at home, and very few sick people were able to receive services in a hospital or clinic setting. From the beginning of the 20th century to its close, hospitals became part of everyday life that were no longer places of sanctuary for those shunned by society. Hospitals became a place for women to bear children, medical specialties to achieve perfection, and new interventions to be proved, as well as a place where nurses cared for those who needed a cure or wanted respite from suffering and pain. By the end of the 20th century, however, patients and families were limited in their opportunities to stay in a hospital, yet this time it was for very different reasons. Common medical

procedures and those services that did
not require extended technological or
medical interventions were now routinely done in the outpatient setting,
where technology was available while
patients were treated. Once surgery
or other procedures were completed
and the patient was stabilized, equipment and monitoring was readily discontinued. Patients then would return
home to finish their recovery. Medical
ideas, values, and morals determined
what hospitals of today would be and
their role in the life of Americans.

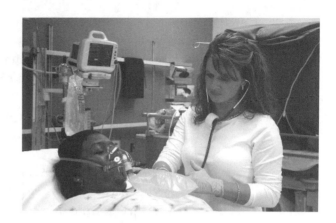

   With limitations in length of stay
and eligibility for hospitalization, there has been a resurgence of home and
community nursing services. A number of very specific home health services have been perfected, such as hospice services, home health nurses for
the elderly, pediatric visiting nurses, and others. They provide an array of
services caring for those who cannot stay in the hospital or who need further nursing or rehabilitative services. Generally, the services of a registered
nurse (RN) are not provided every day around the clock; their visits are episodic (scheduled or on demand), so
patients who require continuous care
are often cared for by skilled nurses
or nurses' aides who are present when
the RN is not.

   About 400 cases of acquired
immunodeficiency syndrome (AIDS)
were diagnosed in a male homosexual
population during 1981; it was later
determined to have been caused by
a new infectious virus called human
immunodeficiency virus (HIV). The
emergence of this contagious disease

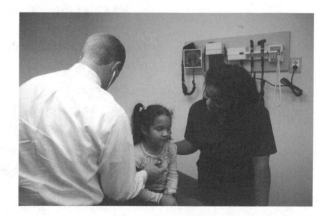

came during an era when many were complacent about communicable diseases, since, in the United States, vaccines had all but eliminated most of the common serious transmittable ones. Discovery of this viral process stimulated research and created national and world health concerns while reinforcing the notion that despite the most sophisticated technologies and knowledge of pathophysiology, there were still many things we did not understand and could not control related to health.

During the last 20 years, accumulated knowledge related to disease management, medical innovations, treatments, interventions, and preventive services have far surpassed anything imaginable. The following are some advances that have transpired:

- Genome studies and a better understanding of genetics and biological markers indicating susceptibility to DNA-linked disease, in vitro fertilization, animal and human cloning, and stem cell research.

- Emergence and identification of new infectious diseases and subsequent advancements in virology and bacteriology. These new strains have significant complications, morbidity, or mortality. Some of these diseases are the result of human behaviors and some are not. This includes the ebola epidemic, resurgence of pertussis, eruption of meningococcal infection in students, drug-resistant strains of tuberculosis, hantavirus infection in New Mexico, mad cow disease and meat contamination, aggressive strains of salmonella and *E. coli* in the food industry, human papilloma virus and cervical cancer, hepatitis C identification (now the most prevalent blood-borne infection), methicillin-resistant *Staphylococcus aureas* in hospitals and other healthcare facilities, appearance of recurrent *Clostridium difficile*, and others.

- Development of routine organ transplantation services, a global network that supports organ recovery for anyone who is eligible, and better technology and pharmacology for optimal outcomes.

- Biomedical research and innovations including pharmacology, imaging, medical waste management, medical informatics, wound and skin care, new and refined surgical techniques (laser-assisted in situ keratomileusis, a variety of scope surgeries, robotics, fluoroscopy, computed tomography guided surgery, and magnetic resonance imaging for surgical intervention), oncology research with novel treatments, and clinical trials for a number of diseases including cancer, hepatitis, and AIDS.

- Disease-specific research and practice recommendations in the areas of stroke, diabetes, hypertension, hyperlipidemia, asthma, chronic obstructive pulmonary disease, atherosclerosis, Alzheimer's disease, Parkinson's disease, depression, osteoporosis, osteoarthritis, rheumatoid arthritis, lupus, heart disease, and other diseases and conditions.

- Advances in recognition, diagnosis, and treatment of mental health diseases, with a significant emphasis on pharmacologic interventions.

These accomplishments and other developments in specialty medicine have continued to change healthcare options while creating numerous opportunities for nurses. Today, nurses can pursue almost any interest they have and acquire skills and knowledge specific to that specialized interest. With specialization has come the rise of certifications and specialty education for nurses as well as other healthcare providers. Advanced practice nurses have also been able to develop practices caring for certain populations by age or by disease category.

War and Its Effects on Nursing

THE MOST RECENT WARS INVOLVING the United States are part of an ongoing conflict in the Middle East. In reality, the current conflict began in 1980 when Iran and Iraq were involved in a dispute as oil prices and oil control became major issues globally. In 1990, Iraqi troops entered Kuwait and war ensued; Iraq gained control of the country in literally 1 day (Donahue, 1996. p. 234). The United States initiated trade embargoes and suspended financial interactions, and the conflict eventually led to the Gulf crisis, Operation Desert Shield, and then Operation Desert Storm. These U.S. offenses were part of efforts from various countries coming together to defend freedom. More women served as combat soldiers, an era of new warfare technology ensued, and there was better international cooperation than in any previous war. As U.S. soldiers and the daily situations of the conflict were brought into the homes of Americans via television, many started to look at war differently; they realized more fully that people served, as well as the implications of that individual effort to secure freedom for all.

Operation Desert Shield led to Operation Desert Storm, and the United States provided the majority of the resources for "the armed force of the Coalition that defeated Iraq, [it] totaled 737,000 men and women ... with 532,000 troops, 120 ships, 1,800 aircraft—thirty four nations provided personnel and equipment in action or in support" (Blair, 1992, p. 125). Thousands of nurses were deployed to Saudi Arabia and other areas of the Persian Gulf region to provide nursing services to male and female combat soldiers or military personnel. During this conflict, American nurses collaborated with nurses from other countries and a global nursing community was formed to serve in an area of the world where women were often oppressed, wore certain customary clothing, and could not be in a public place without a male escort. Nurses once again showed great courage and stamina as they not only cared for those who were sick or wounded, but concerned themselves with those around them in war-torn communities.

Nurses were sent to desert sites

> ... to get ready for a job [they] hoped [they'] never have to do ... they put together "hospitals" from tents to serve as first-aid stations. In battle, crews of RNs and techs would work close to the scene of action, keeping men from bleeding to death and pushing oxygen and IV fluids. Once stabilized, the wounded would be transported to field hospitals. In the field hospitals, those trained to deal with trauma patents awaited their arrival. The Gulf crisis necessitated the use of active duty nurses and reserve nurses, throughout this war and the Afghanistan conflict that would follow, more reserve military personnel were utilized than ever before. As hospitals throughout the nation responded to the call-up, there was concern over how they would deal with the situation and how long it would last. ("Headline News," 1990)

Many nurses were still deployed as the Spirit of Mercy project and other similar programs brought hope and Christmas to nurses who never expected to see the world this way (Sears, Duden, Loughney, & Pruchniak, 1991, p. 26).

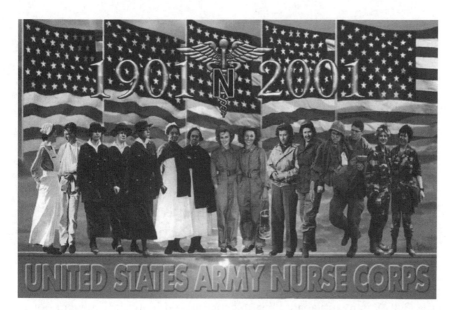

United States Army Nurse Corps, 1901-2001

In 2001, a few weeks after terrorists attacked the World Trade Center and the Pentagon, more reserve nurses and doctors were called into service as U.S. military action in Afghanistan escalated. War nurses participated in caring for the wounded, the sick, and the emotionally distressed individuals who were casualties of the battles that ensued. Some individuals have reported symptoms associated with diseases and syndromes that could have been caused by low-dose, repetitive exposure to chemicals or toxins. There are continued efforts to prove the existence of chemical warfare due to these reports. Health problems associated with explosive devices have caused significant injury, blood loss, and amputations for many. These injuries will continue to cause many to suffer long after they have left the battlefield. Many nurses worked on hospital ships equipped with frozen blood and plasma, monoclonal antibody treatments for large wounds, an extensive array of antibiotics, innovative trauma technology and surgical suites, and improved antichemical remedies (Donahue, 1996).

Elusive symptoms appeared in many who participated in these encounters; those who fought during the first Persian conflict in the early 1990s with continued unexplained symptoms have been identified as having

Persian Gulf syndrome. Epidemiological studies were initiated by the Veterans Affairs Office, Department of Defense, and other research institutions to clarify the causes of this phenomenon. As troops and nurses remained overseas, health and wellness became an issue even for medical providers; issues and challenges were associated with sanitation, waste disposal, endemic infectious diseases, exposure to toxic substances, environmental conditions such as the extreme heat, and emotional and psychological effects of prolonged deployment. Many needed further support when they returned home with physical and psychological problems, including posttraumatic stress syndrome. It is unclear just what the United States will need to do to deal with these health concerns; in the short term, funding has been provided by Congress to allow those who need services to get them. Veterans hospitals and military clinics have expanded services, and more nurses will work with these veterans in the future (Hyams, Riddle, Trump, & Wallace, 2002). As more veterans return from the conflicts that have happened since the Gulf War, unanticipated health concerns (both physical and emotional) will continue to arise.

Nursing Workforce Issues

A N AGING POPULATION, WHICH IS the result of better healthcare options and innovations, has created a need for healthcare alternatives. Skilled nursing homes, retirement communities, and assisted-living residences have appeared in many communities, and these facilities have generated a need for nurses and others to care for their patients. The Social Security Act has prohibited the use of government funds for this type of service, and so the medical assistant or nurse's aide has usually cared for this needy population. Since there are limited financial incentives for extended healthcare facilities and for the professionally trained nurse in such a setting, pay is generally very low and the work very demanding for anyone who works in such an organization.

Implications of the aging population are not fully understood, yet in the short term, many healthcare providers will be required to care for them. Specialty healthcare areas have focused on their needs, and many programs have been initiated to deal with this population. Nurses will have opportunities to care for them in a variety of settings. Of great concern is the fact that Social Security and Medicare benefits are expected to cease or at least decrease significantly during the next decade because expenditures far exceed revenues. Already, nurses are presented with challenges in caring for the aged as Medicare benefits are changed. Patients now have to pay more out-of-pocket expenses, and on their fixed incomes, some choose between food and medical care, particularly related to their pharmacologic needs. In a society where many elderly people are not cared for by their extended families, there will be issues concerning how to care for these individuals and the potential increased need for assisted living and rehabilitative services.

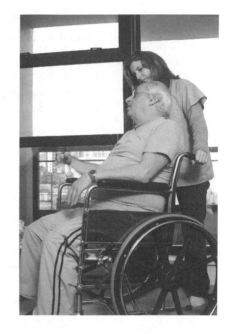

There was an increase of over 400% in the number of employees needed to care for the elderly in nursing homes across the Unites States from 1960 to 1980. Prior to 1980, nurse's aides comprised about 45% of these employees while another 10% were licensed practical nurses, and only about 7% were actually RNs. There were major changes in employee populations at most facilities annually, adding to problems of quality and continuity of care (Kalisch & Kalisch, 2004, p. 433). Of great concern were aspects of patient care, including the following: (1) opposing pharmacological agents ordered and given; (2) patients not routinely followed by attending or facility physicians; (3) orders outdated or not renewed; (4) patients' medications not monitored for interactions; (5) lack of specific monitoring related to administration and response to treatments or medications; (6) lack of adequate patient hygiene or nutritional support; (7) patient infections and/or skin ulcers; and (8) unqualified personnel providing the majority of care routinely.

Most facilities from 1980 until 2000 had a managing RN who generally was unable to provide direct patient care because managing RNs were required to supervise and plan patient interventions. If they did work in the role of a floor nurse, they were often responsible for administering medications to all of the residents or patients. The absence of a qualified licensed nurse was the reason for so many issues associated with nursing home care. Because Medicaid supplements some care in nursing homes, there have been some federal studies undertaken to assess the situation and to make recommendations.

With little funding available for this type of nursing care, along with the need to keep costs to a minimum, unskilled caregivers have provided most of the care on a daily basis. Thus, appropriate skilled care became an issue that prompted nurses and other organizations providing care for the aged to petition for better nurse–patient ratios and regulations on the number of unskilled personnel who could care for this important and vulnerable population. The debate on this issue continues to be a major problem today. Many states have now determined that unlicensed assistive personnel and medical aides certified can assume certain nursing roles in order to care for this population.

Through medical and technological advancement, nurses became the primary providers of patient care. During the 1990s, significant questions were raised related to entitlement of care, and "consumer expectations … values of individualism, competition, cost containment, efficiency, and technology …" became the driving forces of healthcare policy and healthcare systems (Donahue, 1996, p. 446). The nation experienced an increasing gap between the rich and the poor, with a middle class that could no longer maintain its current lifestyle status. The result of this shift in economics meant that many could no longer receive health services that had once been considered a universal right. Questions relative to life and death arose, including who is eligible to receive lifesaving care, lifesaving organs, expensive therapies, experimental treatments or medications, and life-sustaining procedures "when not [everyone] can? Will the rich, the elderly, and the poor receive quality, if not equal care? How and by whom will decisions be made?" (Donahue, 1996, p. 446).

Until the 1990s, 90% of all healthcare expenditures were paid for by insurance companies, Medicaid, or Medicare (third-party payers). As inflation slowed, healthcare costs continued to rise and reasonable cost reimbursement was no longer acceptable. Healthcare reform was initiated and the roles of all nurses, including those of the advanced practice nurse, changed in ways that caused many to wonder about quality of care, which had always been a priority for nursing. With the introduction and establishment of diagnosis-related group (DRG) reimbursements, hospital stays shortened and health care began an evolutionary return to community and home nursing services.

The development of defined outpatient services became one mechanism for administering services with a more economically sound outcome. As these surgical and specialty care clinics evolved, nurses left the hospital to care for patients in these alternative centers. With the advent of these types of patient services, health care became more of a for-profit industry.

Bulger (1988) appealed for a balance of governmental control and healthcare resources:

> There are three strands in relation to the American system of health … a reintegration of technology, bureaucracy, and healing into a new, more humane, and more effective approach to health care. [The postmodern paradigm] would preserve liberty, freedom, hope, and a sense of human progress which incorporates suffering and death, all united through a sense of belonging and community. (pp. 86–87)

By the mid-1990s, many were without healthcare coverage, others were underinsured, and even those who were insured had rising premiums for basic services and interventions. Reimbursement for surgical interventions, expensive diagnostic tests, and other medical treatments were approved and deemed medically necessary by the third-party payers and not by the medical providers who had knowledge and medical expertise related to patient care. Throughout the nation, many programs were devised and initiatives undertaken to control cost containment. Two ideas that in reality were polar opposites when it came to nursing roles and duties emerged. One strategy for success was cross-training of nurses to do many tasks that perhaps others had done previously; for example, labs were drawn by nurses and intravenous (IV) lines were placed by the floor or emergency room nurse rather than the IV team. This concept took nursing toward a primary nursing care model, where the nurse cared for just a few patients who she would follow during their entire stay. Another strategy placed more emphasis on professional tasks that could only be performed by the nurse. Ancillary teams such as respiratory therapy began to provide services that nurses had previously performed to free time for nursing treatments and interventions so that nurses did not do things that others could do. Thus nurses returned to some of the traditional floor models that were similar to the medication or treatment nurses, who were responsible for a larger number of patients with focus on just a few professional nursing duties.

In any case, looking at the bottom line became the focus of many health-care organizations, and their decisions ultimately affected nursing care as assistive personnel and specialty service caregivers replaced nurses on the floor. Innovative ideas prompted changes in the length of shifts, shift combination options, and shift groupings, and a variety of new work environments became available for the individual nurse to consider. Nurses could work in the hospital, in a surgical center, in a subspecialty clinic, in a school, in the community, in home health, in hospice, in a primary care clinic, or in any number of outpatient treatment facilities. With waning hospitalizations, nurses also had many options outside the traditional acute care setting. Despite this diversity, however, in acute care settings, the typical patient acuity rose, and nurses cared for patients with multiple problems and complications in a shorter period of time. In most hospital settings, intensive care units became focused on a particular body system or a category of diseases; for example, there were cardiac or cardiovascular intensive care units, cardiothoracic intensive care units, neurology or neurosurgical intensive care units, and so on. Moreover, many hospitals have specialty floors aside from the general medical or surgical units where nurses focus on a particular set of problems, interventions, and educational strategies to promote best patient care.

For the first time in many decades, healthcare issues arose from preventable diseases associated with lifestyle and affluence. These new concerns, along with new infectious diseases, complicated issues associated with nursing care. Many patients were treated for complications of chronic and interrelated diseases such as hypertension and stroke, or diabetes and hyperlipidemia. As a result, many specialty units and outpatient care centers focused on health concerns of advancing disease rather than on preventive health strategies, since Americans still believed that they were entitled to a quick fix or cure. As these interventional services became more perfected, there arose a need for services outside the hospital that focused on alternative methods of healing and curing. By the end of the 1990s, these types of services were expanding, and nurses had even more options when they considered what practice setting fit their individual nursing goals.

Many inactive nurses returned to work to supplement family incomes, and as they were socialized back into nursing there were generational issues, mentoring dilemmas, and educational barriers that had not been recognized before. Ideas and concepts associated with each generation needed to be addressed in order for nursing to become a cohesive unit that could progress into a more professional future, while still meeting the demands of a global nursing community. Over time, reactivated nurses gained confidence and acceptance in the various settings where they worked. However, with considerable importance placed on higher educational standards and continuation of education, nurses who were educated long ago and nurses who were more recently educated encountered challenges as new ways and old ways came together. Since medical technology is ever-expanding, the new must replace much of the old when it comes to pharmacology, interventions, and understanding of disease.

Licensure and Regulation

LEGAL RESTRICTIONS AND REGULATIONS ARE determined by the individual states of the nation. Nurse practice acts describe the various roles of nurses related to their educational preparation and their corresponding scope of practice. This is important because nursing autonomy and advanced practice models have changed what nurses are legally prepared to do. They define rules and regulations of practice based on common law (social morals, common sense, principles of reason, and accepted justice) and legal law (written regulations related to discipline, authority, competency, unsafe practices, etc.). These nurse practice acts protect the public's interest while maintaining standards of competency for anyone who is licensed.

Nursing has great need for autonomous regulation of the discipline; increased specialization has allowed nurses to practice in areas never before available to them. With the rise in specialty care, many nursing organizations have been founded to support nurses who practice in a specific area of focus. The American Nurses Association developed a national credentialing center, the American Nurses Credentialing Center, which certifies that nurses have met minimum standards in a specialty area and are considered capable experts within the constraints of their practice. They have also been instrumental in promoting magnet status to facilities that promote safe and positive environments for nurses while satisfying the 14 forces of magnetism.

These forces of magnetism identified and adopted by the American Nursins Credentialing Center (2008) include:

1. Quality of Nursing Leadership
2. Organizational Structure
3. Management Style
4. Personnel Policies and Programs
5. Professional Models of Care
6. Quality of Care
7. Quality Improvement
8. Consultation and Resources
9. Autonomy
10. Community and the Healthcare Organization
11. Nurses as Teachers
12. Image of Nursing
13. Interdisciplinary Relationships
14. Professional Development

Other specialty groups related to specific nursing interests have also developed certifications that are recognized nationally, the American Academy of Nurses and the NLN are two groups that administer tests and grant national certification to those who complete all requisites and pass the test. The NLN continues to administer the national RN test as well as the practical nurse test. Once an applicant has passed these exams, he or she is eligible to apply for licensure and work as a new graduate nurse in any facility in which he or she is qualified to work. With these programs, the public is protected and the profession controlled efficiently.

Nursing Research

THROUGH THE EFFORTS OF THE Division of Nursing Research, nursing research was encouraged to develop conceptual frameworks specifically for the discipline of nursing. Once most nursing programs were associated with academic institutions, nursing was required to show that it had a scientific basis. Because nursing was considered an art, the caring aspects of the practice required descriptions. The Division of Nursing Research supported educational opportunities for the profession at the national level and eventually recommended the establishment of the National Institute for Nursing Research. It became affiliated with the National Institutes for Health and the national organizations promoting standardization of nursing education. Emphasis was placed on completion of a master's degree, advanced practice roles for nurses, and faculty development. Various nurse training acts prior to this time were extended under Title VIII, allowing for both faculty and student researchers to receive grant funding for their projects. An almost endless effort by nurse researchers, educators, and students resulted in a substantial amount of published and unpublished research that has changed nursing practice and provided the body of knowledge to support evidence-based practice in any setting.

Nurse theorists continued their work and many more conceptual frameworks have been developed since the beginnings of nursing theory during the 1960s and 1970s. Nurses of today have many theories to support the science of caring and nursing. These theories define nursing and nursing applications in primary care activities, specialty care activities, preventive care, community care, outpatient services, and disease-specific nursing interventions.

> The evolution of nursing has occurred within a political context that has placed many constraints upon the developmental process … In this context, doctoral education for nurses and in nursing is but another step in the overall struggle for independence and recognition. Doctoral programs [place] an emphasis on the methodologies and knowledge base necessary … in basic scientific disciplines upon which the science and art of nursing rest. (Grace, 1978, p. 114)

Extensive studies of nursing, of specific interventions, of nursing functions, and of outcomes have validated nursing theory, the art of nursing, and the science of nursing.

Summary

SINCE THE 1980s, MAJOR CHANGES in health care affected access to care and eligibility for care and have left the nation in a healthcare crisis. Reform was a topic associated with the presidential election in 2008. Despite significant strides in all areas of medicine, discussions about who can and will receive medical services will be forthcoming. Changes in revenue have not only affected care related to DRGs, but have impacted all social government programs. Medicare and Medicaid have had several fiscal cuts decreasing allocation of funds to both the young and the elderly populations. As previously indicated, there is great concern over the viability of these programs in the future and the resultant dramatic fiscal implications.

Innovations and biomedical advances have prompted several new areas of medical care. With the advent of these specialized procedures, nursing specializations evolved and eventually required credentialing and regulation. Nursing roles have been transformed, and nationally there has been enhanced education, regulation, and certification as responsibility, accountability, and opportunity are delineated while protecting nursing autonomy and practice.

Nurses desire to be considered professionals, yet the media and implications of perceived image seem to be an issue for them once again. Nurse researchers have continued to validate the profession as one that is based on theoretical science, cognitive ability, technical skills, and the art of caring in ways which allow the RN's interventions and interactions with the patient to impact and change outcomes as they care. Nurses will need to portray the image that they desire through actions and words.

⬙ IDEAS FOR FURTHER EXPLORATION

1. Review current ideas about healthcare reform. What considerations are there to ensure access to care for all? Reflect upon what you remember about early nurse leaders and their attempts to bring health care to the people.

2. Assess the implications of a multigenerational nursing workforce. Describe one or two characteristics of each generational category and one or two issues that might be present in a nursing unit because of those characteristics.

3. Choose an area of specialty care that interests you (i.e., nurse anesthesia, oncology, etc.). Briefly research and discuss how nursing in that

area of practice has changed with recent certifications and the formation of specialty care nurse associations.

4. What effects have DRGs had on nursing care in the United States?

✦ DISCUSSION QUESTIONS: APPLICATION TO CURRENT PRACTICE

1. Changes in education were implemented over time in order to advance the practice of nursing. What NLN or American Nurses Association recommendations are still in effect today? How do these affect curriculum or student experiences in the age of technology?
2. Cultural competency is considered necessary in the healthcare arena. How can this be accomplished? By whom? What might you do to minimize and/or eliminate cultural bias of gender, ethnicity, or generation in the workplace among your peers or patients as you practice nursing?
3. How can nurses improve their image today? Explain your answer using examples. Identify and describe three strategies for improving the image of nursing that might be helpful for today's nurses.

✦ MeSH SEARCH TERMS

Ambulatory care facilities
Clinical nursing research
Diagnosis-related groups
Gulf War
Iraq War, 2003-

National Institute of Nursing Research
Nursing staff, hospital
Persian Gulf syndrome
Private practice nursing

✦ SUGGESTED READING

Cox, C. W. & Hale, J. F. (2008). *Nurses' experiences in war and disaster: Lessons learned and needs identified.* Philadelphia: Saunders.

Figueroa, D. (2002): *The most qualified: A nurse reservist's experience in the Persian Gulf War.* New York: Vantage Press.

Ivanov, L. L. & Blue, C. L. (2008). *Public health nursing: Leadership, policy, & practice.* Clifton Park, NY: Delmar Cengage Learning.

Kassner, E. (1993). *Desert Storm journal: A nurse's story*. Lincoln, MA: Cottage Press.

Malka, S. G. (2007). *Daring to care: American nursing and second-wave feminism*. Urbana: University of Illinois Press.

Ruff, C. L. & Roper, K. S. (2005). *Ruff's war: A Navy nurse on the frontline in Iraq*. Annapolis, MD: Naval Institute Press.

◈ REFERENCES

American Nurses Credentialing Center (2008). *Forces of Magnetism*. Retrieved June 29, 2008, from http://www.nursecredentialing.org/Magnet/ProgramOverview/ForcesofMagnetism.aspx

Apold, S. (2008). The doctorate of nursing practice: Looking back, moving forward. *The Journal for Nurse Practitioners, 4*(2), 101–108.

Blair, A. H. (1992). *At war in the Gulf: A chronology*. College Station: Texas A&M University Press.

Brinkley, A. (2003). *American history: A survey* (11th ed.). New York: McGraw-Hill.

Bulger, R. J. (1988). *Technology, bureaucracy, and healing in America: A postmodern paradigm*. Iowa City: University of Iowa Press.

Cohen, S. (2007). The image of nursing: How do others see us? How do we see ourselves? *American Nurse Today, 2*(5), 24–26.

Donahue, M. P. (1996). *Nursing: The finest art* (2nd ed.). St. Louis, MO: Mosby.

Grace, H. K. (1978). The development of doctoral education in nursing: A historical perspective. In N. L. Chaska (Ed.), *The nursing profession: Views through the mist*. New York: McGraw-Hill.

Headline news: Military nurses rally for Operation Desert Shield. (1990). *American Journal of Nursing, 90*(10), 7, 11.

Houweling, L. (2004). Image, function, and style: A history of the nursing uniform. *American Journal of Nursing, 104*(4), 40–48.

Hyams, K. C., Riddle, J., Trump, D. H., & Wallace, M. R. (2002). Protecting the health of United States military forces in Afghanistan: Applying lessons learned since the Gulf War. *Clinical Infectious Diseases, 34*(Suppl 5), S208–S214.

Kalisch, P. A., & Kalisch, B. J. (2004). *American nursing: A history* (4th ed.). Philadelphia: Lippincott, Williams, and Wilkins.

Sears, A., Duden, J., Loughney, J., & Pruchniak, J. L. (1991). Nurturing nurses in the Persian Gulf. *American Journal of Nursing, 91*(4), 26.

Spratley, E., Johnson, A., Sochalski, J., Fritz, M., & Spencer, W. (2001). *The registered nurse population, March 2000: Findings from the national sample survey of registered nurses.* Merrifield, VA: Health Resources and Services Administration, Information Center.

CHAPTER

10

Envisioning the Future of Nursing

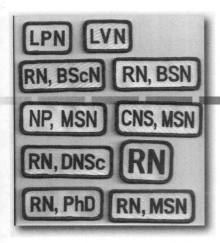

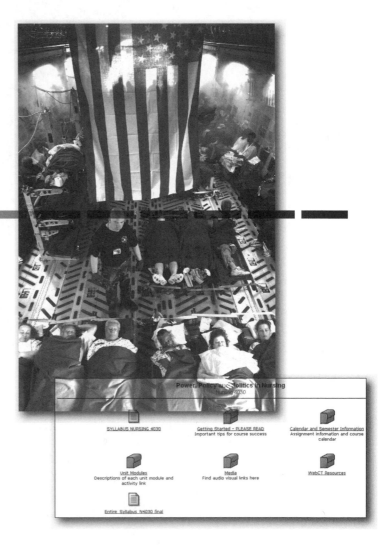

GLOBAL NURSING, NATIONAL HEALTHCARE REFORM, AND NURSE SOCIALIZATION

Deborah M. Judd

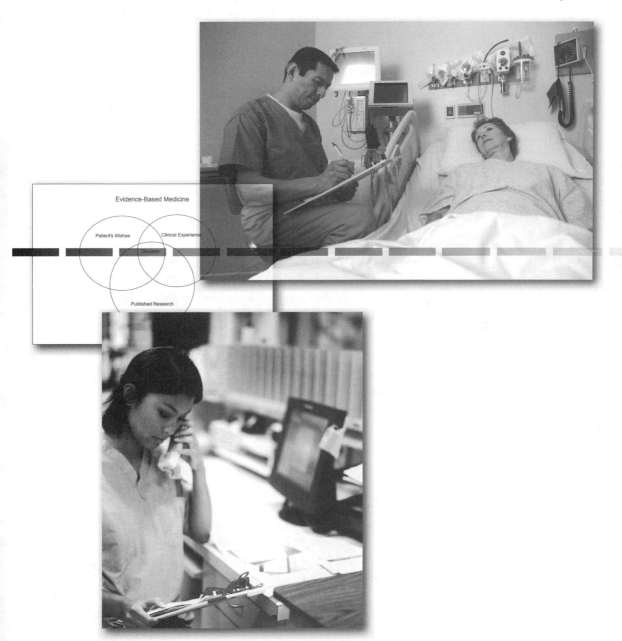

Sociopolitical Climate

THE ELECTION OF 2008 WAS an historic one, as citizens of the United States were given choices never before available. Who should lead our nation? Senator Barack Obama was the first African American candidate nominated by a major political party, and Senator Hillary Clinton, who, if elected, would have become the first female U.S. president. Obama and Clinton were supported by various Democrats, while Senator John McCain and Governor Mitt Romney vied for the Republican Party's nomination. Governor Romney eventually withdrew from the race because of issues associated with his religious background. McCain chose Sarah Palin as his vice presidential candidate; prior to this election, women and minorities had participated in candidacy campaigns, but they had never become serious contenders as these candidates did.

During the entire campaign, a number of interesting accounts emerged on all of the candidates. At times these caused distress for the public as the campaign issues became entrenched in negative publicity and tactics. The election issues really were concerns from the public about the ability of the candidates regardless of who would be chosen to lead the homeland and determine policy related to healthcare reform, economics, and the war. The campaign revitalized interest in politics, and groups of citizens who might not normally participate became involved. On November 4, 2008 Obama was elected President of the United States, ushering in an era of anticipated change.

Global issues still abounded; there were concerns over continued presence in Iraq, worry over oppression in many countries, unease over fuel prices, apprehension regarding involvement of the United States in regional disputes, and fear of terrorism. At the same time there were efforts to promote collaboration in the interest of economics, human rights, world trade, and humanitarian efforts. The country became less self-indulgent as the nation responded to world events with generosity, unity, and commitment. As a result of the economic crises in the United States, the national economy changed and its stability was in jeopardy.

Closer to home, a number of social matters had Americans worried. There were huge numbers of uninsured or underinsured, health care was in need of reform, and social programs of the past were facing huge deficits and overexpenditure. Immigration issues were prevalent, drug problems rampant, nontraditional families continued to emerge, violence was more widespread, and prisons were filled to capacity. Mental health disease was not adequately cared for, women were often the victims of crimes that were perpetrated by those they knew, homelessness was problematic for many communities, and child or elder abuse was not uncommon. Health disparity and access continued to plague the nation, and there were pleas for health-care reform.

This nation of prosperity developed a number of health issues related to lifestyle. Obesity became an epidemic, and with it increased prevalence of common chronic diseases associated with extra weight, unhealthy diets, and sedentary lifestyles. Adolescents and children are now affected; recent statistics suggest that about 14% of children ages 5–8, 19% of school-aged children, and 17% of adolescents are obese. Today almost 70% of all adults over the age of 64 are obese. Overall about one third of the nation would have a diagnosis of obesity based on the standard body mass index (BMI) of equal to or greater than 25. BMI is calculated using the following formula:

$$BMI=kg/m^2$$

However, it is generally determined using reference tables (United States Department of Health & Human Services, 2008; Jordan-Welch & Harbaugh, 2008). Smoking accounted for many health concerns, and efforts funded by the Tobacco Settlement continued to decrease its incidence in hopes that concomitant diseases would be better controlled. Epidemics of diseases associated with risky behaviors have continued to be problematic, the incidence of human immunodeficiency virus (HIV) has decreased in the United States but is still a global issue, and hepatitis C has become an epidemic. Many healthcare resources have been utilized to combat theses infectious diseases and others that have emerged. In addition, the frequency of mental health problems has escalated.

America has become a nation with more immigrants and refugees than ever before. The slogan "the melting pot" has taken on a whole new meaning. According to the Center for Immigration Studies, 11.2 million people immigrated to the US during the 1990s, and from 2000 until 2007, an additional 10.3 million immigrants arrived (Camarota, 2001; Camarota, 2007). Because so many people have arrived in the United States during this relatively short period of time, there are a number of social issues not so very different from those of a hundred years ago . Health care and how to deliver it, not only to those citizens born here but also to those who have naturalized or noncitizens who have sought refuge, is one of the issues nurses will face as they care for diverse individuals in a number of settings. To deliver "essential services to the people of the world, particularly underserved populations, the transformation of the nursing profession is critical, and professional nurses must assume roles as leaders and active participants in change." (Simms, 1991, p. 37). Nurse leaders today will need to look back to nurse leaders of the past, their role models, and take a stand as many of them did to ensure liberty and happiness. The United States will continue to be a leader in determining objectives and strategies with international health partners.

The Image of Nursing

NURSING IN THE 21ST CENTURY changed dramatically as registered nurses worked in every aspect of acute and long-term care; they managed and operated public, industrial, and community health departments, and they achieved diverse skills and specialization of practice. Nurses who continued their education gained advanced degrees and enhanced their nursing roles. They are now nurse practitioners, clinical nurse specialists, nurse educators, nurse researchers, nurse administrators, and nurse legislators—all of whom became examples for nurses entering into the profession and for those who will follow them.

Lavalle (2006) described ways that nurses might improve their image in "Ten Things You Can Do TODAY to Enhance Nursing's Image." Nurses must be self-confident and present themselves as proud to be the registered nurses they are. They should be in charge as they prioritize patient care and keep track of the situation in whatever manner works for them. Nurses who are really professionals do "not just work [their] shift, but embrace [their] work [being] the brightest and the best." She advises that nurses not be "the nurse that everyone hopes isn't working today" (p. 18). Nurses should be involved and know what is going on around them; be familiar with their patients yet not forget peers are there, too. Nurses should take care of themselves so that they can take care of others. They should find someone they would like to mentor or encourage into the profession. Nurses shouldn't be afraid to laugh; there is enough sadness and stress in the day and they should not forget to thank other nurses for what they do (Lavelle, 2006).

In 2004, the American Association of Nurses and the Center for Nurse Advocacy introduced the RN patch as way for nurses to identify who they were. The Center for Nurse Advocacy designed and promoted the RN identification patch so that patients would be able to tell who was the nurse. The embroidered patch was a simple and innovative approach to the problem. It was not expensive and still allowed for individual or unit choice about what type of scrubs on which it would be placed. The pro-

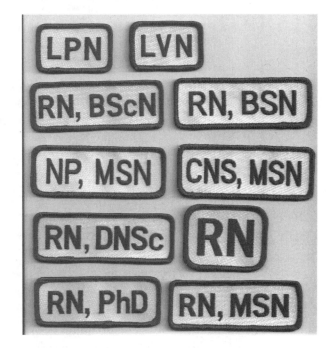

RN patches

moters believed this was an "elegant solution to nursing's identity crisis" at the time (Mason & Buhler-Wilkerson, 2004, p. 11). The plain RN patch was developed by J. Morgan Pruett & Mark Dion, and was introduced by the Center in the April *American Journal of Nursing*.

The Center for Nursing Advocacy is a nonprofit group determined to change the image of nurses as portrayed in the media. Their desire is to promote the profession positively while correcting misrepresentation of and inaccurate information about nurses. They have run several campaigns to dispel inappropriate nursing stereotypes, myths about practice, and connotations about servitude, as well as prevent marketing strategies that represent nurses in a sexualized or naughty manner or as a quack. The center has effectively changed media portrayal of nurses on a number of occasions since 2002, and will continue to promote the profession and improve the public's image of nurses into the future.

The Education of Nurses

NEWMAN DESCRIBES A PROFESSIONAL DISCIPLINE as being "defined by social relevance and value orientations ... derived from a belief and a value system about the professional's social commitment, the nature of service, and responsibility for knowledge development" (as cited in Andrist, Nicholas, & Wolf, 2006, p. 163). Nurse educators must determine a way to enable nurses to know how to apply the science of nursing to the application of nursing. Cody (as cited in Daly et al., 1997) feels that many nurses complete an entry-level degree with only technical knowledge and lack further leadership and cognitive abilities necessary for the profession to grow. There is a gap between what students learn and what they need to understand and be able to do. At entry into practice, they do not comprehend nursing phenomena sufficiently to be able to provide discipline-specific care (Fawcett, 2000). "Emphasis on theory and research in mainstream education often does not concern ... discipline specific-research." (Andrist et al., 2006, p. 167). If the discipline of nursing is to succeed and be recognized, students will need to be prepared to contribute to the profession. They should not be trained to just merely obtain the minimum for licensure, which is often viewed by academia as entry into an occupation. Since nurses are not rewarded for their educational achievements through salary or role description in many organizations, some believe that the technical nurse is equivalent to the Bachelor of Science in Nursing (BSN) nurse.

In order for nurses to be considered professionals, nursing must meet the requirements for a profession. Leddy and Pepper (2006) list the accepted characteristics of any profession (Box 10-1). Nursing does meet most of these characteristics; however, the debate over extensive training and education is not yet resolved. Most other careers considered a profession require a bachelor's degree or higher for entry into practice and credentialing (Leddy & Pepper, 2006). Barger (2006) suggested that the following characteristics define a profession: (1) expert knowledge; (2) autonomy; (3) governance; and (4) service to society. Expert knowledge leads to autonomy and governance. As nurses continue to pursue advanced degrees and validate the science of nursing through discipline-specific research, they will be able to define the nursing profession more effectively (Barger, 2006).

Box 10-1   Professional Characteristics

- ❏ Authority to control its own work
- ❏ Exclusively unique body of knowledge
- ❏ Extensive period of formal training
- ❏ Specialized competence
- ❏ Control over work performance
- ❏ Service to society
- ❏ Self-regulation
- ❏ Credentialing systems to certify competence
- ❏ Legal reinforcement of professional standards
- ❏ Ethical practice
- ❏ Creation of a collegial subculture
- ❏ Intrinsic rewards
- ❏ Public acceptance

Source: Adapted from Hood, L. J., & Leddy, S. K. (2006). *Leddy & Pepper's conceptual bases of professional nursing* (6th ed.). Philadelphia: Lippincott, Williams, & Wilkins.

Patricia Benner described nursing roles in her book, *Novice to Expert*, where she defined 10 specific roles of nurses and the process of becoming an expert nurse. Of course, practice makes perfect, or nearly perfect, and over time one becomes more expert in critical thinking skills, technical skills, and ways of knowing. An experienced nurse can and does achieve some knowledge that is considered equivalent to concepts and components of a BSN education. Despite this fact, should nurses who entered into practice with an Associate Degree in Nursing (ADN) be considered a technical nurse or a professional nurse?

The following synopsis is based on Benner's ideas related to role development and eventual expertise, which come from both academic experiences as well as workplace opportunities. She states that as **caregivers**, nurses nurture and provide; as **colleagues**, nurses provide support for their healthcare peers (especially nursing peers); and as **client advocates**, they do much to promote the best care and/or cure for their patients. As **teachers**, nurses inform others of the rationale for treatments, the choices they have related to treatment, the process of diagnosis and treatment, and other aspects of care. Nurses teach those things that validate the patient and family holistically. They teach in almost every interaction (Benner, 1984).

She goes on to say that as **counselors**, nurses listen and respond to all the needs of patients and provide support for each individual because he or she is a unique person. As **critical thinkers** nurses utilize the nursing process, which allows them to make nursing diagnoses and devise treatment plans since they practice autonomously. Nurses are better than most at determining problems and providing solutions; it is thus that their voices count so much in political and organizational arenas (Benner, 1984).

Benner continues by explaining that nurses are **change agents** and **coordinators** who advocate for their patient's best interests. Nurses know the patient and understand much about his or her challenges and needs. Because of this, nurses can be effective in collaborating with others. Nurses' roles as **administrators** include delivering and monitoring treatments and medications and participating in nursing councils to improve practice. Some nurses ultimately function as nurse administrators, promoting best nursing practices, and becoming **advocates** for nursing, health care, and nursing's future. All nurses can be advocates by enlightening others about the

Evidence-based practice

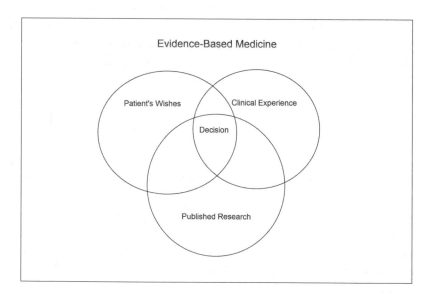

profession, healthcare issues, and nursing issues, and therefore can be nurse professionals, nurse citizens, and perhaps nurse activists (Benner, 1984).

Students should be educated on how to utilize evidence such that their interventions are guided by appropriate evidence-based practice. They also need to understand how to incorporate knowledge and practice guidelines in such a way that they can overcome barriers in the workplace, such as lack of leadership, motivation, vision, strategy, and direction among nurse managers since in most institutions there is a gap between research and application (Ciliska, 2006).

Nurse socialization is an area of education that should be addressed as more and more nurses are affected by multigenerational character- istics and institutional characteristics. It is a well-known fact that nurses eat their young—not literally, but at times they do not care for each other as they should. Since all nurses are needed, or they would not have been hired, nurses must be cognizant of how they accept new nurses who are new graduates, reentry nurses, or nurses who are making a change in their area of practice. They must develop mentoring programs that will provide satisfaction as nurses enter a new unit or organization since retention and recruitment are affected by this. Nurses may have a tendency to act the vic- tim and to backbite or complain, but this is not professional behavior and should be eliminated. If problems or concerns arise, there are better ways to handle them.

Educational programs should mentor students on healthcare policy, organizational policy, and professionalism. Policymakers want to know what nurses think and what the issues are related to nursing, health care in general, and patient care. Beverly Malone, president of the National League for Nursing, advised nurses to remember the nursing shortage we experi- enced 30 years ago; nurses were able to influence Congress to grant funds for education through a nurse training act. Our current nursing shortage will require the same commitment and will not be successfully alleviated unless we deal with the issue of the current shortage of nursing faculty. It is estimated that by 2025, the nation will need 500,000 more nurses than will be available. Who will educate them? The American Association of Col- leges of Nursing agrees that more and more qualified prospective students will be unable to enter nursing because there will be no one to teach them. Both of these organizations encourage nurses and students to make their voices heard. Title VIII is something that nurses need to advise legislators to continue supporting so that the predicted nursing crisis can be eased (American Association of Colleges of Nursing, 2008).

Opportunities for students are changing; there are many new approaches to education that will change the way nurses are prepared in the future. Many nursing programs now have distance learning options, online classes, hybrid classes, and face-to-face classes. Clinical experiences can be gained in a variety of ways. For basic clinical experiences, students still spend many hours practicing hands-on skills in the clinical practice lab or with patents directly in the hospital, nursing home, or clinic. Computer technology has enhanced clinical experiences through a variety of different learning methods and sensory encounters. Students can listen to heart sounds on a DVD or a computer; they can see anatomy via digital photographs or virtual images, or by hands-on experiences in a cadaver lab. Others will interact with simulated patients in very real and lifelike circumstances in simulation labs or self-teaching modules. Students of the future may face choices related to how they learn and meet the outcomes of the courses required. Some students will be able to define elements of their clinical experience to meet personal and program goals. Online courses, hybrid courses, virtual classrooms, webcasts (individual learning modules), podcasts, webinar groups, telenet classrooms, and face-to-face instruction are a few of the current options for students. With continued improvement of technology, creative teaching strategies will emerge to enable students and faculty to exchange information and allow for adequate nurse preparation. Already,

Online nursing course

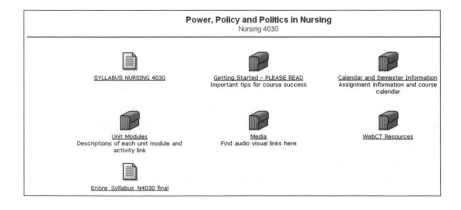

students in one state can take courses at a campus in another state without ever literally being there.

The National League for Nursing (NLN) has continued to promote quality nursing education in the constantly changing worlds of education and health care. This organization has defined educational and clinical practice guidelines for students and educators. The new millennium has brought challenges concerning how to educate and where to educate future nurses and nurses choosing to advance their education. The NLN has recommended educational guidelines and outcomes for nurses at all levels, from the practical nurse to the DNP. There are initiatives for technology and innovation in nursing education, creative educational models, and strategies for how to educate multigenerational nurses. The NLN also has promoted a new certification for nursing professors, the Certified Nurse Educator (CNE). In 2008, the NLN instituted a nurse educator program to incorporate and implement the newest technology and teaching strategies into the classroom. A selected group of nurse educators will participate and become experts who can coach peers as they adopt new ways of instructing nurses. Finally, along with monitoring educational standards, the NLN continues to provide testing services in order for nurses to become licensed (NLN, 2008).

Advances in Nursing

THERE ARE LIMITLESS POSSIBILITIES RELATED to biomedical developments. Each and every day there are many new insights, some minor and some major. The human body is no longer a mystery, and even in the last 20 to 30 years, medical knowledge has increased significantly. With this knowledge, many innovative strategies will materialize and continue to change the way medicine is practiced and the care nurses will provide. The basics of hygiene and sanitation should remain in the forefront of infectious disease management, and utilization of hand sanitizer and hospital-wide hand-washing programs will continue to be effective despite new ideas and discoveries in that particular field.

New and better techniques for diagnostic and procedural imaging will change the way many patients are treated. Robotics and other electronic endeavors may revolutionize care as human contact decreases for procedures and intensive care units. Computer technology has already changed the way we detail interventions, electronic medical records are the future of documentation, and they will be perfected such that documentation in any system will eventually be linked. The options are unlimited in how nurses can manipulate that data to effect best patient care and outcomes. The linkage of information from any system or pharmacy will allow patients to be most effectively cared for as all aspects of their health maintenance are considered.

Pharmacology advances are an almost daily occurrence as medications are altered or developed to treat almost any condition. Many of the new drugs are active metabolites, decreasing side effects and increasing bioavailability. With diseases that present major problems for society or the individual, rules and regulations granting FDA approval have been revised so that those who need the medications can get them more easily and perhaps more readily.

War and Its Effects on Nursing

A T THE TIME THIS BOOK publishes, the nation will still be involved in regional war efforts. Many do not support the administrative decisions that entered the country into these conflicts or agree with the reasons it is still involved in the disputes. Meanwhile, nurses continue to serve in the military, performing nursing tasks and responsibilities as they care for those far from home who require their services. They have served in difficult circumstances during all wars and have been revered generally for that which they have done. With technological innovations, it is likely that warfare will continue to change and that nurses will be required to learn and adapt to the unique medical conditions that may come from nuclear or chemical warfare while still providing services necessary for trauma, burns, and surgery to repair damaged bodies.

Nurses follow troops into unfamiliar regions and circumstances that may necessitate new technical skills and perhaps better interventions for emotional and mental challenges that are prevalent in such arduous conditions. It is anticipated that chemical and biological warfare will escalate and that targets of war may no longer be the enemy, but the civilians of the enemy's society.

Mass causalities could occur if infectious agents such as anthrax or other potentially lethal viruses or bacteria are used. Viral warfare may be more difficult to manage since there are limited options for treatment. Contamination of water sources might become a problem if communities are the target. Terrorism may become a method of war that will be very difficult to manage; the enemy can be at home rather than only on the battlefield. Patients may not be the typical soldier but rather nonmilitary patients who have by no choice of their own been in the path of destruction. If that is the case, wartime patients may be young or old, complicating care since there are unique health matters specific to each group in the life span.

As methods of combat associated with new aircraft prototypes, unmanned vehicles, and robotic activities are developed, nurses will care for patients in a much different way. If robotics progress, the nurse might or might not be present with a patient. Remote facilities are now in trials throughout the country, and

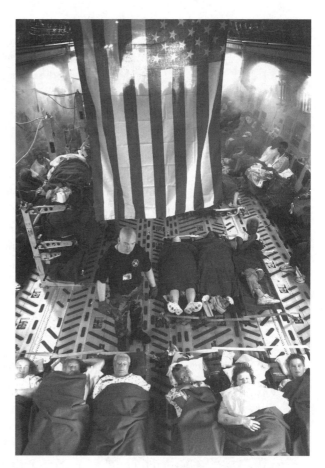

Flight Nurse Captain Gary Hardy helps prepare to transport sick and injured Hurricane Katrina victims

currently only a handful of nurses or technical support personnel are in attendance. Doctors and specialists can render care remotely as the patient is managed through monitoring devices that allow for care options based on technical information and orders from wherever the doctor might be.

More subtle and devious methods, such as emotional or psychological distress, may be prevalent in wars of the future. One author believes that the media could present challenges for governments waging war (and in turn, for nurses caring for patients) based on its reporting.

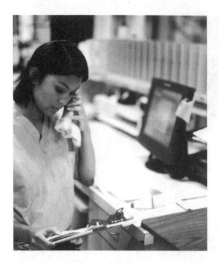

Governments that wage future wars will find that the public support they depend upon is more likely to waver if graphic images are screened of, for example, the massive civilian casualties that may eventuate during such a campaign. As a result they are more likely to cave into public pressure in an act that amounts to a "half-measure"—one that mixes all the disadvantages of a military strike with all those of having done nothing at all. (Howard, 2003)

Such portrayal could also sway public opinion on the help that nurses are providing. Although nurses serve in wars, it is important to remember that their objective is to provide care for the wounded and ill, and their presence does not necessarily indicate their support of the war itself.

Nursing Workforce Issues

NURSES TODAY HAVE A VARIETY of opportunities because of the efforts of many nurses from the past. Countless nurses have devoted their lives to the profession; others have worked tirelessly to provide health care required no matter what the situation or the circumstance might have been. Numerous nurses made choices as did Florence Nightingale to reach beyond themselves as they sacrificed aspects of daily life in order to achieve dreams that would allow nurses to better themselves and the profession. Nightingale felt that individual nurses and the profession of nursing as a whole would facilitate changes into the future, changes that she did not personally see. Nurses would eventually understand how to provide best care to ensure maximum recuperation or to facilitate an optimal death. (Nightingale, 1860). Nightingale stated that:

> No system can endure that does not march. Are we walking into the future or into the past? Remember we have scarcely crossed the threshold of uncivilized civilization in nursing: there is still much to do ... In the future, which I shall not see, may a better way be opened? May the methods by which every sick person will have the best chance of recovery, be learned and practiced! (as cited in Donahue, 1996, p. 417)

Despite great strides in practice and professionalism, there are still issues that have not been resolved, and concerns about them require nurses to come together to assess and evaluate their challenges while planning and implementing strategies for their solutions. Nurses are wonderful as they use this process, the nursing process determined and described by them, in all aspects of their lives, especially in the role of a nurse.

> In order to advance the discipline toward the future, the new tomorrow, nurses have to unite themselves in an effort to construct new organizational and legal structures and thus bring more clarity to their roles as professionals. They can no longer allow others to do the job for them ... within the context of "Health for All" movement nurses [will need] to redirect their attention from primarily hospital care [back] ... to the sick in the community. ... [Is] the discipline ready to accept this challenge with competence ... [taking] on [the] role as a pathfinder [instead of] waiting for directions [to be] given by other disciplines, who are often less well equipped to act as a liaison between the policy-makers and planners of care and the public at large? (van Maanen, 1990, p. 922)

Nurse migration is likely to create concerns as women with increased mobility choose to come to the United States in search of something better; they are interested in better pay, better working conditions, career mobility, professional development, a better quality of life, personal safety or sometimes just novel adventure (Kingma, 2006). International recruitment is believed by some to be the answer to the nursing shortage; however, others believe that retention of nurses is a better way to manage the shortage and correct the underlying issue. Dissatisfaction, lack of prepared nurses and faculty to prepare them, poor wages or benefits, mandatory overtime, high patient acuity, staffing ratios, and callback or call-off policy are the issues that should be addressed to keep nurses from leaving the profession (Kingma, 2008).

There are more male nurses today than ever; they account for about 5% of the registered nurse population in the United States. Many of them practice in critical care areas and often continue education, enabling them to labor in the advanced practice areas of nursing. They generally practice as nurse anesthetists, nurse practitioners, nurse educators, and nurse managers if they have completed a master's degree or higher. Those with a baccalaureate degree often work in acute care in the critical care, trauma,

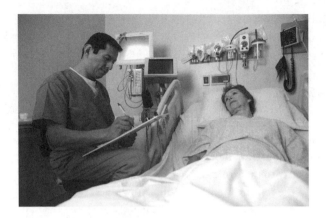

or emergency room units. A recent national campaign has promoted male nurses in order to change the public's perception of them. This campaign was sponsored by the Johnson & Johnson Company and used the catchphrase, "Are you man enough to be a nurse?" This effort has helped the image of male nurses, allowing them to be more readily socialized into nursing by their peers and to be better understood by the public. In the movie *Meet the Parents*, the male nurse is queried about when he will become a doctor. This stereotype actually still exists; often the male nurse is mistaken for the doctor or patients wonder if he is in school to become a doctor.

A unique approach to nursing is required; the nurse who is the primary caregiver for the patient in the hospital or who assists the family in the community setting must advocate for that patient individually and for all patients collaboratively to promote ultimate recovery (Donahue, 1996). They will have to acknowledge that because of increased responsibility, extended autonomy and knowledge, they have an obligation to serve self, the profession, and humanity. Some of the professional challenges they face as they have entered the 21st century are:

1. Issues associated with their working environment and work conditions

2. Staffing, patient acuity, and nurse-to-patient ratios

3. Salary and benefits

4. Practice standards, role definitions and delineation of responsibility

5. Frustration with ability to provide best care in the current healthcare arena, which features cost containment and insurance determination of care, unlicensed assistive personnel, lack of cooperation, etc.

6. Barriers to autonomy and decision making

7. Concerns over image and lack of unique identity

8. Difficulty using acquired knowledge and decision-making ability

9. General public lacking knowledge about what a nurse is and what she or he does—determined in part by media portrayal

10. Apparent lack of concern related to legislation, lobbying, and support of professional organizations

11. Diversity and specialization

12. An impending nurse shortage, lack of adequate nursing faculty, nursing school acceptance quotas too low for the significant prospective applicants, and lack of funding for nursing education

13. Continued dispute over educational requirements to define the entry level of practice

14. Multigenerational differences

15. Multicultural challenges—patients and peers

It might appear that there are more questions to be answered than there are answers to them. If one were to browse recent online bulletins sent out by the American Nurses Association, one would find headlines such as the following:

- Nurse leaders to end racism
- Residency program gives graduate nurses confidence
- Nurses join profession at midcareer
- Case managers to coordinate care
- Hospitals create brighter environment
- N.Y. nurse shortage brings higher salary
- Men choose nursing for intrinsic value
- Nursing programs add costs to students
- Nurses take action to protect workplace violence
- Ailing U.S. economy may ease the nursing shortage

One would also find success stories about mandatory overtime, safe staffing victories, and revamping nursing education.

Licensure and Regulation

LICENSURE AND REGULATION WILL CONTINUE to evolve such that nurses nationally will abide the same standards. The professional organizations that now help to regulate educational standards, educational degrees, and national testing will continue to do so in the future. Their influence on curriculum will allow for nursing students to receive consistent information as they meet standardized criteria at any level of preparation. Licensure remains the best way to maintain control over establishing capable and competent nurses. Regulation of practice should still be determined by individual states but must be legally defined in a similar manner throughout the entire United States. As a global nursing community develops, regulation may even be needed at an international level, especially in light of nurse migration.

Educational level will continue to be debated, yet nurse practice acts determine the entry level of practice in each respective state. As has been done already in some states, the baccalaureate degree is legally defined as the educational entry level for a registered nurse. Due to frequent nurse shortages, there will always be a place for other levels of nursing, but will those levels considered to be more technical and will they still have the same licensure or credentials in the future?

The American Nurses Association (ANA) has continued to protect the profession of nursing through a variety of programs. This organization is very involved in policy and standards of practice. They have developed a nursing code of ethics, defined nursing rights, and become the premier credentialing agency for nurses. The American Nurses Credentialing Center (ANCC) promotes nursing excellence through continued education and enhanced practice opportunities. The ANCC has developed the Magnet Recognition program, which encourages organizations that employ nurses to provide a safe and encouraging environment in which nurses can work towards certification.

The ANA created the National Database of Nursing Quality Indicators (NDNQI)® to enhance nursing practice and determine areas where organizations and nurses can improve quality of care. The indicators measured in the quality evaluation process include: falls, falls with injury, nursing care hours per patient day, skill mix, pressure ulcer prevalence, and hospital-acquired pressure ulcer prevalence (Montalvo, 2007). There is also an optional survey that can be administered to assess nurse satisfaction and issues of relevance in a particular organization. As these indicators and nurse satisfaction continue to be assessed, further recommendations related to practice standards, licensure, and credentials will be made. It is anticipated that this quality promotion program along with the Magnet Recognition program will encourage cooperation and advance the profession through credentialing and recognition of excellence.

Nursing Research

RESEARCH WILL CONTINUE INTO THE future as nurses describe assessment, interventions, and outcomes. Publications and Web sites offer access to a wealth of information on a variety of topics and specialties. As more and more nurses and institutions search for articles and recommendations relevant to their area of nursing care delivery and expertise and then apply those standards, nursing care will change as they document the interventions and their outcomes. A search of any database will produce thousands of articles on a variety of nursing subjects. But what does the profession do with that body of knowledge?

There may be some questions such as: Who is this knowledge for? Who needs to know it? Do all nurses in a given facility need to see it? Who is accountable for disseminating it? How does it affect the responsibility of advanced practice nurses? These questions are still unanswered, yet there are some thoughts about them. Perhaps certain clinicians would accept the responsibility to review and share relevant literature (research) with those who could benefit from it the most. Clinical nurse specialists and other advanced practice nurses might be the most appropriate ones do so. Other nurse managers might be involved as they develop protocols relevant to their units for evidence-based practice (EBP). This is necessary in light of our litigious society, where all nurses will be held accountable for standards of practice specific to general patient care but more specifically to diseases and to procedures they perform, even if they personally have not seen those guidelines.

Thus, it is the responsibility of all nurses to remain current in their practice through continuing education and affiliation with specialty organizations or nurse educators in their respective organizations. As always, documentation is extremely important: if it is not documented, it is not done. If patient status and interventions are missing, nurses may be at risk. The ANA has promoted standards of practice, and many specialty or subspecialty nursing groups have based their practice protocols on those basic nursing practice guidelines. The ANA has even developed specific standards, expectations, and scopes of practice for each RN role. As nurses continue to become expert in very specific nursing roles, there will be a need to define these roles further, including level of autonomy and credentials for practice.

As educational opportunities continue, nurses will be involved in research. There will be others who are prepared to develop theories, to participate in research, to design studies, and to document outcomes. "One of the highest priorities for creating an appropriate future for nursing is that of identifying, structuring, and continuously advancing the knowledge that underlies the practices" of what we do daily as we care for patients through scientific knowledge and intuitive practices (Cody, 2006). When individuals acquire knowledge, they are determined capable and responsible through examination, licensure, or certification. They should be able to identify, verify, structure, and continuously update their armamentaria in order to be considered a professional (Andrist et al., 2006, p. 287).

Newman (2003) uses an analogy of the World Wide Web to describe a world of no boundaries. Access is unlimited and not dependent on time, location, or situation. Nurses have that same opportunity as they view patients, fluctuations in physical functioning occur over time, in various situations, and in various locations in a rhythmic phenomena. Reality is no longer so complex, but in reality things are

> interwoven aspects of multiple phenomena ... there is no gap between you and your experiences ... this brings us to where we are in nursing knowledge—a world of no boundaries ... a temporal perspective, reality in the present, not what went before, or comes after. (Newman, 2003, p. 242)

Nurses can then describe what it is they see, what it is they do, and what it is that happens. This knowledge then can influence the actions of others as they care for patients in the unique ways that only nurses can.

Summary

THE REVIEW OF NURSING HISTORY has shown us that in all eras, nurses have chosen the profession knowing full well in advance the demands, the issues, the possibilities, the challenges, and the rewards. The quest for the title of registered nurse requires courage, commitment, stamina, flexibility, intelligence, charity, patience, and determination. In the early years, a handful of committed and determined women initiated changes that have allowed nursing to become what it is today. During the years that followed more and more nurse leaders emerged, and even though many of their names are unknown, their contributions have not gone unnoticed as nurses today reflect upon the heritage that they have.

Great opportunities and challenges will always accompany this honorable profession as it continues to influence the lives of so many. Nurses understood their position in the early decades of the 1900s, as evidenced by this public health nurse joke: "A patient asked the nurse if she didn't think that it was nice weather. 'I don't know,' the nurse replied, 'you had better ask your physician'" (Baer, D'Antonio, Rinker, & Lynaugh, 2002, p. 346). Even then they knew the answers, but they also understood their role and responsibility. Today nurses would know the answer to that question and many others; they would tell the patient the things he needed to know to care for himself as he achieved a balance between illness and health. They would care for that patient in ways that only a nurse can. They would use cognitive skills, technical skills, interpersonal skills, spiritual skills, psychosocial skills, and emotional skills as they practice with autonomy and responsibility.

✤ IDEAS FOR FURTHER EXPLORATION

1. Learn more about nursing issues and concerns by completing an internet or periodical search. You may use the topics from the ANA SmartBrief list in this chapter and/or find some of your own. List one to three topics and briefly describe what is being done to alleviate or correct the problem. Go to nursingworld.org and find current nursing concerns and options for you to join SmartBrief or other free ANA student services.

2. Review the NLN (http://www.nln.org/), ANA (http://www.nursing-world.org/), or Center for Nursing Advocacy (http://www.nursingadvocacy.org/news/news.html) Web sites. Discuss what you have learned and how the organization is working for nurses nationally.

◈ DISCUSSION QUESTIONS: APPLICATION TO CURRENT PRACTICE

1. What is a discipline? How will nursing be able to show that nurses are professionals and that nursing is indeed a discipline? Share examples.
2. Educational approaches are changing. What types of educational opportunities exist for students? How do these affect the way nurses are prepared? Explain how student needs and issues are being addressed. Give specific examples.
3. How can nursing intervene to alleviate the predicted nursing shortage? How will the healthcare professions deal with this? Give examples and relate them to scope of practice, authority, responsibility, or competency.

◈ MeSH SEARCH TERMS

Computer simulation

Computer-assisted instruction

Decision making, computer-assisted

Diagnosis, computer-assisted

Healthcare reform

Insurance, health

Lifestyle

Managed care programs

Medical informatics

Medicare

Obesity

Patient simulation

Surgery, computer-assisted

Telemedicine

◈ SUGGESTED READING

Barger, R. N. (2006). *Characteristics of a profession*. Retrieved March 28, 2006, from http://www.nd.edu/~rbarger/profession.html

Benner, P. (1984). *From Novice to Expert: Excellence and Power in Clinical Nursing Practice*. Englewood Cliffs: Prentice Hall.

Cherry, B. & Jacob, S. R. (2008). *Contemporary nursing: Issues, trends, & management.* (4th ed.). St. Louis, MO: Mosby Elsevier.

Camarota, S. A. (2000). *Census Releases Immigrant Numbers for Year 2000.* Retrieved September 1, 2008, from http://www.cis.org/articles/2002/censuspr.html

Camarota, S. A. (2007). *Census Releases Immigrant in the United States, 2007.* Retrieved November 4, 2008, from http://www.cis.org/articles/2007/back1007.html

Cohen, M. H. (2003). *Future medicine: Ethical dilemmas, regulatory challenges, and therapeutic pathways to health care and healing in human transformation.* Ann Arbor: University of Michigan Press.

Grossman, S., & Valiga, T. M. (2005). *The new leadership challenge: Creating the future of nursing* (2nd ed.). Philadelphia: F.A. Davis.

Nursing's agenda for the future: A call to the nation. (2002). Washington, DC: American Nurses Pub.

Montalvo, I. (2007). The National Database of Nursing Quality Indicators (NDNQI ®). Online *Journal of Issues in Nursing, 12*(3).

Sullivan, E. J. (1999). *Creating nursing's future: Issues, opportunities, and challenges.* St. Louis, MO: Mosby.

Weaver, C., Delaney, C. W., Weber, F., Carr, R. (2006). *Nursing and informatics for the 21st century: An international look at practice, trends, and the future.* Chicago: Healthcare Information and Management Systems Society.

Yoder-Wise, P. S., & Kowalski, K. (2006). *Beyond leading and managing: Nursing administration for the future.* St. Louis, MO: Mosby Elsevier.

⚬ REFERENCES

American Association of Colleges of Nursing. (2008). *Nursing shortage resource.* Retrieved August 25, 2008, from http://www.aacn.nche.edu/media/shortageresource.htm

Andrist, L. C., Nicholas, P. K., & Wolf, K. A. (Eds.). (2006). *A history of nursing ideas.* Sudbury, MA: Jones and Bartlett.

Baer, E. D., D'Antonio, P. D., Rinker, S., & Lynaugh, J. E. (2002). *Enduring issues in American nursing.* New York: Springer.

Barger, R. N. (2006). *Characteristics of a profession.* Retrieved March 28, 2006, from http://www.nd.edu/~rbarger/profession.html

Camarota, S. A. (2000). *Census Releases Immigrant Numbers for Year 2000.* Retrieved September 1, 2008, from http://www.cis.org/articles/2002/censuspr.html

Camarota, S. A. (2007). *Census Releases Immigrant in the United States, 2007.* Retrieved November 4, 2008, from http://www.cis.org/articles/2007/back1007.html

Ciliska, D. (2006). Evidence-based nursing: How far have we come? What's next? *Evidence-Based Nursing, 9,* 38–40.

Cody, W. K. (2006). Philosophical and Theoretical Perspectives for Advanced Nursing Practice (4th ed.). Sudbury, MA: Jones and Bartlett.

Daly, J., Mitchell, G. J., Toikkanen, T., Millar, B., Zanotti, R., Takakashi, T., et al. (1997). What is nursing science? An international dialogue. *Nursing Science Quarterly, 10,* 10–13.

Donahue, M. P. (1996). *Nursing: The finest art* (2nd ed.). St. Louis, MO: Mosby.

Fawcett, J. (2000). The state of nursing science: Where is the nursing in science? *Theoria: Journal of Nursing Theory, 9*(3), 3–10.

Hood, L. J. & Leddy, S. K. (2006). *Conceptual bases of professional nursing* (6th ed.). Philadelphia: Lippincott Williams & Wilkins.

Howard, R. (2003). The dangers of warfare in a media age. *The National Interest,* April 23, 2003. Retrieved August 28, 2008 from http://www.inthenationalinterest.com/Articles/Vol2Issue16/vol2issue16howardpfv.html

Jordan-Welch, M., & Harbaugh, B. L. (2008). End the epidemic of childhood obesity one family at a time. *American Nurse Today, 3*(6), 25.

Kingma, M. (2006). *Nurses on the move: Migration and the global health care economy.* Ithaca, NY: IRL Press.

Kingma, M. (2008). Nurses on the move: Historical perspective and current issues. *OJIN: The Online Journal of Issues in Nursing, 13*(2).

Lavalle, A. (2006, August–September). Ten things you can do today to enhance nursing's image. *Modern Nurse,* 18–19.

Mason, D. J., & Buhler-Wilkerson, K. (2004). Who's the RN? Identifying nurses simply by the patch. *American Journal of Nursing, 104*(4), 11.

Montalvo, I. (2007). The National Database of Nursing Quality Indicators (NDNQI ®). Online *Journal of Issues in Nursing, 12*(3).

National League for Nursing (NLN). (2008). *About the NLN.* Retrieved November 4, 2008, from http://www.nln.org/aboutnln/index.htm

Newman, M. (2003). A world of no boundaries. *Advances in Nursing Science. 26*(4), 240–245.

Nightingale, F. (1860). *Notes on nursing: What it is and what it is not.* New York: D. Appleton & Company.

Simms, L. M. (1991). The professional practice of nursing administration. *Journal of Nursing Administration, 12,* 37.

United States Department of Health & Human Services. (2008). *Obesity.* Retrieved August 27, 2008, from http://health.nih.gov/topic/Obesity

van Maanen, H. M. T. (1990). Nursing in transition: An analysis of the state of the art in relation to the conditions of practice and society's expectations. *Journal of Advanced Nursing, 15*(8), 914–924.

CHAPTER 11

Information Technology and the Continued Study of Nursing History

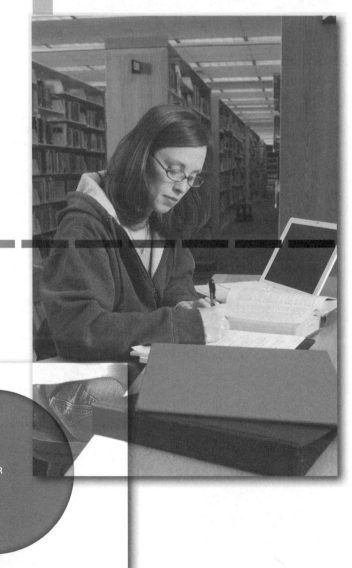

This Venn diagram illustrates results when searching for *nursing*, *war*, and *nursing and war*. Connecting keywords with *and* will retrieve fewer results than searching with a single keyword.

NURSING AND WAR

RESEARCH TIPS AND RELEVANT RESOURCES

G. Megan Davis

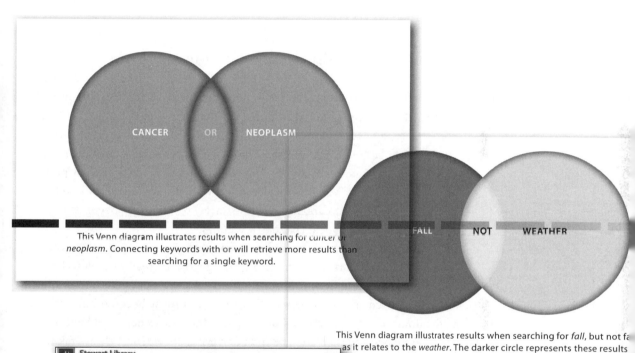

This Venn diagram illustrates results when searching for *cancer or neoplasm*. Connecting keywords with *or* will retrieve more results than searching for a single keyword.

This Venn diagram illustrates results when searching for *fall*, but not *fall* as it relates to the *weather*. The darker circle represents these results. Items that have both *fall* and *weather* will not show up in search results. This search will retrieve fewer results than if the search includes *fall* as a single keyword.

T HE PREVIOUS CHAPTERS HAVE IDENTIFIED key events, people, and trends related to the history of nursing in the United States. The focus of this final chapter is to provide skills and resources to help students conduct their own historical research.

How to Find and Access Historical Information

A S HAS BEEN DETAILED IN previous chapters, nursing research focused on the results of current nursing practice. Research included "studies of nursing practice, nursing services, nursing service administration, nursing education, and the individual nurse ..." (Kalisch & Kalisch, 2004, p. 385). Even this type of research was not undertaken early on in nursing history. The first scholarly journal, *Nursing Research*, did not appear until the early 1950s (Kalisch & Kalisch, 2004). The research conducted and then published in journals such as this was looking ahead, not looking back into the past. Over the last 30 years, however, historical research has become more popular in the nursing field (Fitzpatrick, 2007).

Conducting historical research is different than performing other types of research many nurses are currently engaged in. Instead of undertaking the construction and administration of a research study in the present, a nurse interested in the history of the profession must become immersed in the documents and artifacts of the past. The researcher must find historical evidence and then analyze and interpret that evidence, always taking into consideration the original context of the source. Research of this nature also requires that the historian understands how their current perspective, including personal and societal biases, might affect the interpretation of the source material (Hacker, n.d.). An important aspect of historical research is being able to paint a complete picture of the time period being studied. This requires that the researcher has a working knowledge of the social, economic, and political factors that were in play at the time (McGann, 1997/1998).

When beginning historical research, the initial idea tends to be broad, as is the case with almost all types of research. Browsing a journal like *Nursing History Review* might be a good place to start when looking for a research topic. However, it is very important to narrow the topic down, both to make the research process itself manageable and to avoid an overwhelming literature search. Doing extensive background reading before beginning an in-depth literature search and review is a useful technique when trying to focus in on a topic. This background research will also help determine whether or not there is enough existing material available, and possibly more importantly, accessible, to allow the nurse to proceed with a particular avenue of research (Burns & Grove, 2001). Whenever possible, the researcher should also try to choose a topic that is interesting to him or her, as this type of research may involve significant costs of both time and money. Chosen topics should "be significant, with the potential to illuminate or place a new perspective on current questions, thus contributing to scholarly understanding" (Lusk, 1997, p. 355).

Historical research typically involves two types of sources: primary and secondary. Primary sources are those resources that encompass first-hand, personal, or eyewitness accounts of an event, usually (but not always) written or published around the time of the original incident. Examples include diaries, interviews, oral histories, manuscripts, memoirs, and autobiographies. Primary source material may be in written, audio, or visual format. In historical research, primary sources should make up a large portion of the source material. Secondary sources are resources that provide views on an event from an outside perspective. Examples consist mainly of written works, including both books (like biographies, textbooks, and other nonfiction works) and periodical articles. More critical than finding primary and secondary resources (discussed later on in this chapter) is evaluating the information that one does find. In historical research, this can be extremely important. According to Liehr and LoBiondo-Wood (2006), both validity and reliability of any documents must be established. Validity or authenticity can be established using external criteria. Is this resource everything it seems to be at first glance? Is it representative of the appropriate time and/or person being researched? Determining validity involves examining the document itself for handwriting samples, as well as ink and paper authenticity. In audiovisual materials, the method of recording should be examined and assessed as appropriate for the relevant time period. If a resource is deemed valid, the reliability must then be determined using internal criteria. This is where the researcher's knowledge of the time period becomes crucial as it relates to the larger context of the individual or event being studied. Understanding the language of the time plays a crucial role in evaluating reliability. In general, a primary source is assumed to be more reliable than a secondary source, but it is important to remember that those who recorded events as they happened were actually recording events as they *remembered* them happening or gave their biased perceptions of what actually happened. Combining primary source material with well-balanced secondary sources is key in the historical research process.

Once a research topic or research question has been decided upon, the searching process begins. Before the researcher dives in headfirst, however, it is important to understand where to look for historical material, and to learn to employ search tips that will increase the efficiency of the literature search. Many nurse researchers have become familiar with some of these methods and research tools, in particular using library catalogs and article databases, but historical research also involves delving into the depths of the many archives and special collections held at universities and other organizations.

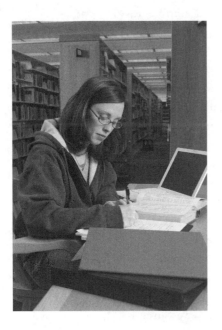

A good place to start, especially when first looking for background information, is the library catalog. Library catalogs contain listings of items held by particular libraries, both public and academic. This can include books, theses and dissertations, and media items. Most library catalogs can be accessed by the public via the library's Web site. (Readers can access the online resources that accompany this textbook for a list of specialty library catalogs, like the National Library of Medicine.) This method can be time consuming since the researcher is accessing one library's catalog at a time and has no idea where relevant materials may be held. A freely available Web resource called WorldCat (http://www.worldcat.org/) is trying to assist researchers in this matter by allowing searching of library catalogs across the world. Here one can type in a few search terms (or an author's name or the title of a work) and see which libraries hold the sought item. Many public and academic libraries provide a service known as interlibrary loan. This service will prove useful if the

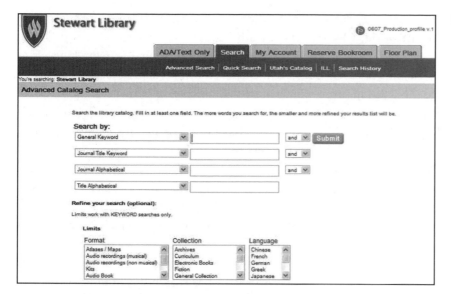

Library catalog

item the researcher is interested in is not available at his or her local library. Periodical articles and books can be requested via interlibrary loan, and the researcher's local library will send inquiries to the libraries that hold the item, asking that it be sent to the researcher. Many library catalogs include items that the library circulates (items that can be checked out) as well as items from their special collections and archives. Most libraries do not circulate materials from these special collections, and thus, they can't be requested via interlibrary loan. In this instance, the researcher will need to contact the person in charge of the special collection or archive and ask if photocopies can be made or if the researcher can make an appointment to visit the collection and see the item in person.

While library catalogs may tell a user if the library subscribes to a particular newspaper, magazine, or journal, they generally do not provide access to the individual articles themselves. For this the researcher needs to become familiar with using a variety of article databases. In the past, researchers looking for periodical articles had to search through print volumes of bibliographic indexes like *The Reader's Guide to the Periodical Literature*. This was extremely time consuming. Now there are a number of useful historical and health-related article databases that are available electronically. These include, but are not limited to, Medline (either the

PubMed or Ebsco interface), the most comprehensive literature database in the world; CINAHL (Cumulative Index to Nursing and Allied Health Literature); HealthSource: Nursing/Academic Edition; Nursing Journals @ Ovid; and JSTOR, a database focusing on historical periodical articles back to the 1600s in some subject areas. With the exception of the PubMed version of the Medline database, none of these article databases is freely available on the Web. Most nurse researchers are affiliated with a clinic/hospital or university that pays for access to these databases. These resources will be available via the institution or university library Web site. The number of full-text articles available differs between institutions based on what the institution or library can afford. Again, interlibrary loans can be used in this instance to request full-text articles from journals to which the researcher does not have immediate access.

When searching a library catalog, article database, or the Web, it is important for the researcher to keep a few search tips in mind. Complete sentences or research questions should never be entered into a search box in any of these tools. The computers that run these searches generally ignore words like *of, the, in*, etc. because they appear in every book, article, and Web site. The researcher should choose several important keywords from the research topic or question and focus on those. Synonyms for these keywords should also be considered, because the researcher does not know which terms various authors may have used. In some instances, the search tool itself provides a thesaurus or list of approved search terms to help guide the researcher in the right direction. In academic library catalogs, this might be the Library of Congress subject headings list. In Medline, this is the medical subject heading (MeSH) list. CINAHL has its own subject headings list as well, similar to MeSH, but not exactly the same. Researchers shouldn't be afraid to play around with these help tools in the library catalog and article databases.

The Web itself can be a great source of information, with a few caveats. First, not everything is available on the Web (for free or even for a fee), which is why library and other institutional collections are so important in the research process. There *are* a significant number of Web resources specifically related to nursing history and historical nursing research. The Web site that accompanies this textbook includes a list of many of these resources. The importance of evaluating resources was discussed previously in this chapter and becomes even more significant when retrieving results from the Web. Anyone can post just about anything online at any time.

When evaluating resources from the Web it is important to consider the following questions: Who is responsible for the content on the site and what is their area of expertise? Is the purpose of the site to inform, persuade, or sell something? Is there some sort of bias involved? When was the site created or last updated? (Note: In historical research, the currency of a site is not as important as it is in clinical research.) Are there sources available to reinforce the accuracy of the content on the site? How much of the site's content is relevant to the research topic?

Once the researcher has chosen keywords and synonyms, he or she can use different ways to connect them to create a search statement, using the Boolean operators: *and*, *or*, and *not*. The default option that is set in most library catalogs, article databases, and Web search engines (like Google) is to automatically connect search terms with *and*, meaning that the search results will include only the items that have all of the search terms in them. This default *and* search does not care *where* those search terms appear in the item, so the search may bring up results that are not exactly useful. In some instances, it matters a great deal where the search terms appear. If the researcher wants to make sure that two or more search terms appear next

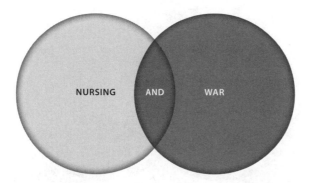

Boolean operator "AND"

This Venn diagram illustrates results when searching for *nursing, war,* and *nursing and war.* Connecting keywords with *and* will retrieve fewer results than searching with a single keyword.

to each in the exact order listed, he or she can enclose the search terms in quotation marks, such as "Florence Nightingale." This is known as phrase searching.

As mentioned earlier, researchers should consider more than just the exact keywords taken from the research topic. Synonyms play an important role in searching as well. The best way to combine synonyms or similar terms in a search is to use the Boolean operator *or*. As the computer reads the search statement from left to right (sort of like a math equation), the terms connected with *or* need to be placed in parentheses so that they will be searched in the right order, such as: ("heart attack" or "myocardial infarction"). Combining synonyms with *or* enables the researcher to retrieve all of the relevant results, regardless of which term or phrase an author used. To avoid missing relevant search terms, researchers can also use the database's thesaurus or subject headings list described earlier in the chapter.

Not is a Boolean operator that is used rarely, but can be very useful when applied correctly. This connector should be used if there is one search term that has multiple meanings, only one of which is relevant to the search. For example, searching for items using the word *Saturn* will bring back results related to both the planet and the automobile manufacturer of the same name. Using *not* as part of the search statement (e.g., Saturn not car) would get rid of the irrelevant results.

Boolean operator "OR"

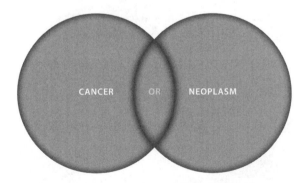

This Venn diagram illustrates results when searching for *cancer* or *neoplasm*. Connecting keywords with or will retrieve more results than searching for a single keyword.

This Venn diagram illustrates results when searching for *fall*, but not fall as it relates to the *weather*. The darker circle represents these results. Items that have both *fall* and *weather* will not show up in search results. This search will retrieve fewer results than if the search includes *fall* as a single keyword.

These Boolean operators are extremely useful when searching library catalogs and article databases, but Web search engines work a bit differently. Most search engines direct researchers to their advanced search pages to construct a similar search statement using text input boxes instead of the Boolean operators themselves. It is a good idea to become familiar with the advanced search features of several Web search engines.

The research tools discussed earlier may be familiar to many who have done research in the past. When undertaking historical research the most important resource that should be considered is an archive or manuscript collection. This is where the historical researcher is going to find the vast majority of primary sources needed to complete a project. Unfortunately, there is no freely available worldwide listing of all of the archives and manuscript collections at all of the institutions throughout the world. As mentioned previously, academic library catalogs are one way to access some of these collections, but a growing number of historical manuscript collections are located outside of the university sphere. This is where using the Web search skills discussed previously can increase success when searching for these mysterious collections. The accompanying Web site provides a comprehensive, though not exhaustive, list of manuscript collections, oral history collections, and archives related to the history of nursing. With the advent of digital technology, many of these organizations are now able to provide online descriptions, and in many cases, images of the items in their collection. Finding aids that describe exactly what that collection holds may be available. Many archival items are grouped together in boxes based on their subject matter or original owner. A finding aid is a list or inventory of the specific items in each box, allowing the archivist and researcher to locate the items he or she is interested in. Accessing these materials is trickier than putting in an interlibrary loan request. At the very least, it means contacting the institution or organization that is in charge of the collection and discussing the research project with someone there. That person might be able to photocopy materials on occasion, but in some cases it will be necessary for the researcher to go to where the collection is held and see the materials in person. This is due to both the fragile nature of many of these primary and secondary resources and the copyright laws governing these collections.

While conducting historical research can be very rewarding, it can also be frustrating at times. In many cases, items have been thrown out before their historical significance was established and they are gone forever. Most institutions and organizations are also forced to base their collection policies on the space that they have available to store these materials and the money they have available to provide upkeep. Some fragile materials must be stored in temperature-controlled environments and must be handled with gloved hands to avoid the oils on human skin. Collection decisions can also be based on the past use of the items. If no one has looked at them for 50 years, they might be the next items to be discarded due to space and budget issues (McGann, 1997/1998).

Contributing to the Discourse: Web-Based Dialogue

THE DEVELOPMENT OF WEB-BASED CATALOGS, article databases, and Web sites has greatly enhanced the research process over the last decade. Other information technologies are helping to augment the ongoing dialogue that nursing research, historical or otherwise, can initiate. There are a number of nursing-specific electronic mailing lists, chat rooms, and message boards that researchers can use to contact others with similar interests. By sharing research ideas and results via the Web, researchers are no longer limited to their own knowledge or that of their colleagues in the immediate area, but can reach out and partake in conversations across physical and cultural boundaries (Pravikoff & Levy, 2006).

Future Directions

HISTORICAL NURSING RESEARCH HAS INCREASED in popularity over the last 30 years, and there are still many directions to be explored. Fitzpatrick (2007) shares some thoughts on possible topics of interest, including the development and evolution of nursing as an organized profession, a scholarly practice discipline, or as a system of education. How does nursing relate to past and current world events? Consider researching controversial nursing figures or techniques. What caused the evolution of one particular technique to another? Nursing history textbooks like this one are a hotbed of historical research ideas.

❖ SUGGESTED READING

See the Web content that accompanies this textbook for a list of print and Web resources related to conducting historical nursing research. This content is available through the publisher's catalog page for this book (http://www.jbpub.com/catalog/9780763759513/), or by visiting www.jbpub.com, keyword "Judd."

❖ REFERENCES

Burns, N., & Grove, S. K. (2001). *The practice of nursing research: Conduct, critique & utilization.* (4th ed.). Philadelphia: Saunders.

Fitzpatrick, M. L. (2007). Historical research: The method. In P. L. Munhall (Ed.). *Nursing research: A qualitative perspective.* (4th ed., pp. 375–386). Sudbury, MA: Jones and Bartlett.

Hacker, D. (n.d.). *Research and documentation online: Researching in history.* Retrieved March 1, 2008, from http://www.dianahacker.com/resdoc/history.html

Kalisch, P. A., & Kalisch, B. J. (2004). *American nursing: A history* (4th ed.). Philadelphia: Lippincott, Williams, and Wilkins.

Liehr, P. R., & LoBiondo-Wood, G. (2006). Qualitative approaches to research. In G. LoBiondo-Wood & J. Haber (Eds.). *Nursing research: Methods and critical appraisal for evidence-based practice* (6th ed., pp. 148–175). St. Louis, MO: Mosby Elsevier.

Lusk, B. (1997). Historical methodology for nursing research. *Image: Journal of Nursing Scholarship, 29*(4), 355–359.

McGann, S. (1997/1998). Archival sources for research into the history of nursing. *Nurse Researcher, 5*(2), 19–29.

Pravikoff, D. S., & Levy, J. (2006). Computerized information resources. In V. K. Saba & K. A. McCormick (Eds.). *Essentials of nursing informatics* (4th ed.). New York: McGraw-Hill, Medical Pub. Division.

Photographic Credits

COVER IMAGES AND CHAPTER 1 OPENER CREDITS   From left to right, beginning at top left: Courtesy of United States Air Force Photo Master Sgt. Lance Cheung, via Wikimedia Commons; Courtesy of the Center for Nursing Advocacy; Courtesy of Dmadeo, Wikimedia Commons; Courtesy of United States Air Force Photo Master Sgt. Lance Cheung, via Wikimedia Commons; Courtesy of the Center for Nursing Advocacy; Courtesy of Dmadeo, Wikimedia Commons; Courtesy of Boston Public Library; Courtesy of the National Archives and Records Administration; Courtesy of Christopher Matta; Courtesy of Man Vyi, Wikimedia Commons; Courtesy of United States Government, Wikimedia Commons; Courtesy of United States Air Force Photo Master Sgt. Lance Cheung, via Wikimedia Commons; Courtesy of Biblioteca del Monasterio de El Escorial, ms T. I 6, fol. 25. Patrimonio Nacional, Spain, Wikimedia Commons; Courtesy of the National Archives and Records Administration; Courtesy of the Center for Nursing Advocacy; Courtesy of Dmadeo, Wikimedia Commons; Courtesy of the Centers for Disease Control and Prevention; Courtesy of Christopher Matta; Courtesy of Biblioteca del Monasterio de El Escorial, ms T. I 6, fol. 25. Patrimonio Nacional, Spain, Wikimedia Commons; Courtesy of the Centers for Disease Control and Prevention; Courtesy of Biblioteca del Monasterio de El Escorial, ms T. I 6, fol. 25. Patrimonio Nacional, Spain, Wikimedia Commons; Courtesy of Boston Public Library; Courtesy of Man Vyi, Wikimedia Commons; Courtesy of the National Archives and Records Administration; Courtesy of the National Archives and Records Administration; Courtesy of Christopher Matta; Courtesy of the National Archives and Records Administration; Courtesy of United States Government, Wikimedia Commons; Courtesy of Dmadeo, Wikimedia Commons; Courtesy of United States Air Force Photo Master Sgt. Lance Cheung, via Wikimedia Commons; Courtesy of the Center for Nursing Advocacy.

CHAPTER 2   *Page 12* Courtesy of Wikimedia Commons; *page 13, top* Courtesy of Biblioteca del Monasterio de El Escorial, ms T. I 6, fol. 25. Patrimonio Nacional, Spain, Wikimedia Commons; *bottom* Courtesy of Sven Dressler; *page 15* Courtesy of Wikimedia Commons; *page 16* Courtesy of the Library of Congress, LC-USZ62-819.

CHAPTER 3   *Page 26* Courtesy of Man Vyi, Wikimedia Commons; *page 29* Courtesy of the Library of Congress, LC-DIG-ppmsca-06809; *page 33* E.B. & E.C. Kellogg and N. York, courtesy of the Library of Congress.

CHAPTER 4   *Page 45* Courtesy of United States Government, Wikimedia Commons; *page 48* Courtesy of Dr. Michael Echols; *page 50, top* Courtesy of the Library of Congress, LC-USZ62-9797; *bottom* Courtesy of the Library of Congress, LC-DIG-cwpb-04246; *page 51* Courtesy of the Library of Congress, LC-DIG-cwpb-01196; *page 52* Courtesy of the Library of Congress, LC-USZ62-90542.

Index

Note: Page numbers followed by an *italicized p* indicate photos; *b*, box.